The Day My Arm Turned Blue

FIGHTING TO BE HEARD AND
FINDING GRACE IN THE STRUGGLE

by Karen "Kay Starr" Smith

The Day My Arm Turned Blue

Fighting to Be Heard and Finding Grace in the Struggle

This book is a work of nonfiction based on the author's personal experiences. In some cases, names, identifying details, and certain circumstances may have been changed to protect the privacy of others.

The information contained in this book is for informational and inspirational purposes only and is not intended to replace medical advice, diagnosis, or treatment from a qualified healthcare professional. Readers should consult their own healthcare providers regarding any medical concerns.

Published by **KindRoot Wellness, LLC**

First Edition

Cover design by Karen "Kay Starr" Smith

ISBN: 979-8-234-05660-3

Printed in the United States of America

Dedication

To my children, Chad and Kaitlyn.

Chad, you have been my steady anchor, carrying responsibilities far beyond your years with quiet strength and grace. Your love has held me up in some of the hardest seasons of my life, and your presence has been a reminder that even in my weakest moments, I was never alone.

Kaitlyn, my beautiful girl, you have been both my reason to fight and my constant reminder of joy. Your laughter broke through the darkest days, your hugs gave me strength when I had none, and your light has carried me through more than you will ever know.

You are my heart, my courage, and my why.

And to every woman who has ever sat in a waiting room feeling unseen, unheard, dismissed, or made to doubt what she knows in her own body, this book is for you.

I carry your stories in mine.

May these pages remind you that your voice is powerful, your pain is real, your story is worthy, and you are never alone.

Acknowledgments

There is no way to tell a story like this without naming the people who helped carry me through it. Chronic illness may happen in one body, but survival is rarely a solo act. This journey has been shaped by the doctors, family, friends, caregivers, and community members who showed up with compassion, consistency, and love when I needed it most.

First, I thank God.

For every breath, every second chance, every answered prayer, and every moment of grace. My faith has carried me through the darkest nights, and I know without question that God's hand has been on my life. His grace held me, His mercy covered me, and His presence never left me.

To my children, Chad and Kaitlyn: Thank you for being my heart outside of my body. Your love, patience, and strength gave me more reasons to keep fighting than you will ever fully know. You have both carried parts of this journey with me, and I thank God every day for the gift of being your mother.

To Cliff and Nikki: Thank you for stepping in and caring for my baby girl when I could not. In one of the most heartbreaking seasons of my life, your faithfulness gave me a peace I cannot fully put into words. Knowing Kaitlyn was safe and loved by people I trusted so deeply meant everything. You helped carry a burden no mother ever wants to lay down, and I will always be grateful.

To Joan: Thank you for loving Kaitlyn so beautifully and treating her as your own. Even with your busy schedule as a gospel singer, you made room for her—taking her to performances across the country and enrolling her in Vacation Bible School. In a season of uncertainty, you provided her with joy and stability. I am certain Kaitlyn inherited her love for singing from you, which makes your influence even more special. Thank you for pouring into her with such generosity.

To Kesta: Thank you for your steady presence through the hardest moments. From hospital stays to emergency room runs, your consistency meant the world—especially when others fell away. Your loyalty and care are gifts I can never fully repay.

To Owen: Thank you for ensuring Chad and Kaitlyn were fed and stayed connected to me during my hospitalizations. Those acts may have seemed simple, but they were monumental. In a season of fear, your kindness brought the comfort and steadiness I couldn't provide myself at the time.

To Stephanie: Thank you for going above and beyond for both Kaitlyn and me. What you did was never just a responsibility; it was love in action. Your tenderness and dependability left a lasting mark on my heart.

To Carol and family: Thank you for loving us during a truly heartbreaking moment. When Kaitlyn was born and I was too sick to leave the hospital, you took my baby girl home and cared for her as your own until I was well. Your selflessness met me in a place of deep pain, and I will never forget it.

To Dr. Patel and your entire team, thank you for being there from the very beginning of this journey. You were the first doctor I saw when my arm turned blue, and in one of the most terrifying moments of my life, you helped save my arm and my life. Thank you for your skill and care through my rib resection, aneurysm repair, stent placements, and multiple clot removals. You gave me hope when I had none, and for that I will always be grateful.

To Dr. Sheira Schlair: Thank you for seeing me, hearing me, and treating me with dignity, compassion, and genuine care. You never treated me like just a diagnosis or a chart to review. You treated me as a whole person, and that meant more than I can ever fully express. Your advocacy, kindness, and willingness to truly listen helped restore a sense of trust in a system that had often left me feeling unseen. You are the kind of doctor and advocate every patient deserves.

To Marjorie (Mommy) and Sonia: Thank you for the kind of love that steadies a mother's heart. Knowing Chad and Kaitlyn were cared for allowed me to focus on survival.

To the medical providers who treated me with respect and humanity: In a system that can often feel cold, your compassion was a lifeline.

And finally, to the readers: To every person who has felt dismissed, unseen, or unheard—this book was written for you. My prayer is that these pages make you feel less alone, more equipped, and certain that your voice matters.

No one gets through a journey like this alone. I know I did not. To everyone who helped hold me up: Thank you.

Table of Contents

Introduction

There are some moments in life that divide everything into "before" and "after."

For me, one of those moments began on an ordinary morning in 2010. I got up to make a bottle for my eighteen-month-old daughter, Kaitlyn, and felt a sharp pain in my left arm. Within minutes, that arm turned blue. I did not know it then, but that moment would become the doorway into a life I never expected. It was a life shaped by blood clots, surgeries, strokes, chronic pain, medical trauma, and a healthcare system that too often made me fight to be heard.

This book was born out of that fight.

It was born in hospital rooms and waiting rooms, out of nights filled with fear, and courage gathered in pieces. It was born from the exhausting reality of having to explain and re-explain my own body to doctors who sometimes listened and sometimes did not. It was born from the heartbreak of being dismissed, the relief of finally finding providers who cared, and the hard-earned lessons of advocating for myself when my life depended on it.

But this book is not only about illness.

It is about motherhood.

It is about faith.

It is about grief and resilience.

It is about what happens when a woman is forced to live inside a body she can no longer fully trust, while still loving, leading, building, and trying to hold her family together. It is about the cost of survival and the grace that grows in the middle of it.

I wrote this book because I know I am not the only woman who has sat in an exam room feeling small. I am not the only one who has left an appointment in tears, or been told it was "just stress" when I knew something was wrong. And I am certainly not the only Black woman who has felt the added burden of having to prove my pain in a system that has too often minimized it.

To those living with chronic illness: I see you.

To those who love them: I hope these pages help you understand the weight they carry.

To the providers: I hope this offers a glimpse into what it feels like to live on the other side of the chart.

This is my story: a story of surviving uncertainty and learning to advocate for a body I felt I had lost. It is a story of pain, yes, but also of purpose. It is a story of children who became my "why" and a faith that held on even when it trembled.

Truthfully, I am still living parts of this story in real time. But I know one thing for certain: silence helps no one.

So, I am telling the truth. I am telling the truth about the battlefield of the body, the loneliness of the hospital room, and the grief of lost independence. I am telling the truth about advocacy, because too many patients are suffering quietly when they should have been taught how to speak.

And I am telling the truth about grace, because even in the middle of the struggle, grace kept showing up. Sometimes it looked like a doctor who truly listened. Sometimes it looked like my son stepping up in ways no young man should have to, or my daughter's laughter breaking through a dark day. Sometimes, it was just one whispered prayer.

If this book does anything, I hope it reminds you of this:

Your body is telling a story.

Your pain is real.

Your voice matters.

This is the story of the day my arm turned blue and everything that came after.

CHAPTER 1

When It All Began

I never expected my journey into the world of chronic illness to begin the way it did.

One beautiful summer morning in 2010, I got up to make a bottle for my daughter, Kaitlyn, who was just eighteen months old. It was such an ordinary moment, the kind of moment mothers live a thousand times without thinking. I had done that routine so many times before. I was still half-awake and moving on instinct with a bottle in hand while my baby girl waited for me. There was nothing dramatic about the morning at first. There was no warning and no sign that life as I knew it was about to change.

I was simply being her mother.

I remember the quiet rhythm of that morning, the small task in front of me, and the feeling of moving through a routine I could do in my sleep. But as I began to wash her bottle, I felt a sharp pain in my left arm. It came suddenly enough to catch my attention, but not yet enough to make me panic.

At first, I brushed it off.

Maybe I slept wrong, I thought. *Maybe I pulled something. Maybe it's nothing.*

But as I kept scrubbing, the pain got worse. It did not happen slowly. It happened quickly and sharply. My arm began to feel heavy and almost foreign, as if it no longer belonged to me. Within moments, it grew weak and useless, dangling at my side. I looked down, and what I saw made fear rise in me so fast that I can still feel it when I think about it now.

My arm was turning blue.

It was not bruised or discolored in some small, explainable way. It was blue. It was the kind of blue that tells you this is not something to wait out. It was the kind of blue that makes your body understand danger before your mind has even caught up. In an instant, the whole room changed. I was no longer just a sleepy mother making a bottle. I was a terrified woman staring at her own arm, knowing something was very, very wrong.

And even in that moment, my first thought was not about me. It was about my baby.

I had a child who needed me. I had to get her dressed, figure out how to get to the hospital, and figure out who would help me. I had only one functioning arm, and pain was shooting through my body, but motherhood does not pause for crisis. When you are a mother, fear and responsibility often arrive in the same breath.

So somehow, through pain and panic, I got Kaitlyn dressed the best I could.

I honestly do not remember every detail of how I managed it. I just remember forcing myself to stay focused while my heart raced. I remember trying not to let my mind spin too far ahead. I remember the fear of not knowing what was happening to me, while also knowing I did not have the luxury of falling apart yet.

I called two of my closest friends at the time, Cliff and Nikki, who were Kaitlyn's godparents. I told them what was happening. They were already on the road, and we arranged to meet halfway so I could hand Kaitlyn off to them. I also asked my upstairs neighbor to drive me, because I knew I could not manage this alone.

There is something humbling about the moment you realize you need help and cannot pretend otherwise.

I have always valued being strong and handling what needs to be handled. But strength looks different when your body is suddenly in crisis. That morning, strength looked like calling people. It looked like asking for help. It looked like doing the next thing, then the next thing, and then the next thing, even while fear was sitting in my chest like a stone.

With one arm limp and in excruciating pain, I handed my baby over to Cliff and Nikki, and my neighbor rushed me to the emergency room. By the time I arrived, everything was moving quickly. The vascular team was called in to examine me, and I could see from their faces that this was serious. After a careful look, the attending vascular surgeon, Dr. Patel, said words that have never left me: "In more than twenty years of practice, I've rarely encountered this condition. This isn't good."

Those words hit hard.

I was already afraid, but hearing a seasoned doctor say that made everything even more real. I pleaded with him the only way I knew how. I said, "Please don't let me lose my arm. I have a baby at home to care for."

Even now, when I think back to that moment, I do not hear my own words as dramatic. I hear them as honest. I was not thinking about vanity or inconvenience. I was thinking about survival, motherhood, and the terrifying possibility that my life could shift in a way I was not ready for.

Dr. Patel promised me he would do everything he could, not just to save my arm, but to save my life.

They discovered a blood clot lodged in my left arm, cutting off circulation and turning my skin that frightening shade of blue. I was rushed into emergency surgery, and by the grace of God, the surgeons were able to save my arm. I thank God for that to this day.

But the surgery was not the end of the story. It was only the beginning.

Recovery was long and painful. I spent weeks in the hospital, separated from my baby girl, while Cliff and Nikki cared for her with tenderness and love. Their presence in that season was a gift I cannot overstate. When I could not mother the way I wanted to, they stepped in and covered us. They made sure my daughter was safe and loved while I lay in a hospital bed trying to understand what had just happened to my life.

There is a particular kind of heartbreak that comes from being a mother in crisis. Your body is failing you, but your heart is still reaching for your child. You are trying to heal, but part of you is still pacing the floor in your mind. You are wondering if your baby has eaten, if she has slept, if she is asking for you, and if she feels your absence. Even when people are helping—and thank God for the people who do help—there is still grief in not being able to do what comes so naturally to you.

I felt that grief deeply. And still, what followed was even more frightening.

After that first surgery, I continued to clot, even while taking medications that were supposed to prevent it. I was prescribed Coumadin, but I clotted anyway. Then I was given Plavix, yet I still had more clots. Other blood thinners were tried, but the clots kept coming. No one seemed to understand why. No one had answers. All I knew was that my body was betraying me, and the doctors did not seem to know how to stop it.

I remember another frightening moment not long after that season began. After a big snowstorm, Kaitlyn and I were sitting in the living room watching a Barbie movie. It was one of those simple moments that mothers hold onto: quiet, ordinary, and full of comfort. But even ordinary moments had started turning on me.

I got up to go to the bathroom and suddenly collapsed to the floor.

My knees would not work. I could not stand. I remember the shock of it and the fear rising fast as I realized my body had once again failed me without warning. I called my friend Kesta and asked if he could take me to the emergency room. The streets were still full of snow and had not been plowed, but he came anyway. He drove through those snow-filled roads to get to me, and I have never forgotten that kind of love.

At the time, Kaitlyn was only about four years old. She had to get herself dressed while all of this was happening. When she came out, her clothes were backwards and all sorts of mixed up, but she had done it. Even now, that memory makes me smile and ache at the same time. She was just a little girl doing the best she could in a scary moment, and somehow that tiny act said so much about the life we were already living.

When I got to the hospital, the doctors discovered that blood was pooling in my knees. The blood thinner that was supposed to help protect me had caused internal bleeding.

It was yet another turn in this already unbelievable journey. It was another reminder that even the treatments meant to help me came with risks of their own. By then, I was starting to understand that chronic illness was not just one crisis or one diagnosis. It was a life of constant adjustments, frightening surprises, and learning how to keep going when the ground under me never felt fully steady.

That kind of uncertainty does something to you. It steals your ease. It changes the way you hear every ache, every pull, and every strange sensation. It teaches you how quickly peace can disappear. In those months, fear became a quiet companion. Every twinge in my arm felt loaded. Every unusual feeling made my mind race. I was trying to care for my children and hold on to some sense of normalcy while privately wondering what emergency might come next.

Then, months later, the real answer came in the most unexpected way.

One day, while I was at home caring for Kaitlyn, I sneezed. It sounds almost laughably small when I write it now: a sneeze. But that sneeze sent a sharp, intense pain through my neck and shoulder. I thought maybe I had strained a muscle, but the pain did not pass. Because of everything I had already been through, I contacted my doctor, who immediately told me to go to the emergency room.

At first, the vascular resident found nothing and was preparing to send me home. That moment could have changed everything in the worst way if not for one doctor who chose to pause. One amazing ER doctor, who knew my history of clotting, insisted on doing an x-ray before discharging me. That decision mattered more than he probably knew. That x-ray revealed something shocking. I had been born with an extra first rib that curved over my shoulder and pressed directly on my left subclavian artery.

A follow-up CT scan showed something even more serious. The extra rib had caused an aneurysm in the artery itself. Finally, there was an answer. The diagnosis was a rare form of Thoracic Outlet Syndrome.

I had never heard of it before. Most people have not. Even many doctors had only read about it in textbooks and had never actually treated a real patient with it. Hearing that left me feeling two things at once: relieved and terrified.

I was relieved because finally I had proof that something real was happening inside my body. I had proof that the clots were not random and proof that I had not imagined the danger. My body had been speaking the truth all along. Yet I was terrified because the answer was rare, serious, and life-threatening.

There is something unsettling about being told that your case is unusual even among professionals. It makes you feel exposed and vulnerable. It feels like you have stepped into territory where certainty is thin and even the experts are learning as they go.

I needed surgery immediately.

The night before the procedure, Dr. Patel tried to lighten the mood with humor. Because it was a teaching hospital, the residents had to get my permission before they could observe or sit in on the surgery. Since my case was so rare, I saw it as a valuable opportunity for these young doctors to learn, so I kept saying yes to every resident who came to ask. Dr. Patel laughed and joked, "If you give permission to one more resident to observe your surgery, there won't be room for you on the table. Please stop it."

I laughed, but underneath that moment was a sobering truth. I was no longer just a patient. I had become a case. I was a rare one whose suffering had become educational to the people around me. And while I understood the value of that medically, it was still strange to realize that the thing threatening my life was so uncommon that it had become something others wanted to study.

The surgery lasted eight hours. They removed the extra rib, repaired the aneurysm, and performed a bypass to restore proper blood flow. It was grueling, but it saved my life.

Looking back now, I realize that this was the true beginning of my health journey. It was not just because of the clot, the diagnosis, or the surgery, but because it was the moment I was pulled into a world I could never fully leave behind. It was a world of specialists, scans, hospital stays, and constant vigilance. It was a world where you learn the geography of your own body through pain and become fluent in urgency.

But the truth is, my health struggles had started even before that day.

When I became pregnant with Kaitlyn, I was already battling serious health issues. Early in my pregnancy, I was diagnosed with congestive heart failure. Most of my pregnancy was spent in the hospital with doctors trying to keep both me and my baby alive. At one point, I sat in the emergency room for nearly forty-eight hours because no unit wanted to take responsibility for me. The cardiac unit was afraid I would go into premature labor, while the maternity ward was afraid my heart would fail.

So I waited, caught in the middle. I was too cardiac for one floor and too pregnant for another. Eventually, I was admitted to the cardiac unit. My baby's lungs were supported with steroids, and by the grace of God, she was born healthy.

So much of my motherhood began under the shadow of survival.

And then, only eighteen months later, I found myself back in the emergency room again. This time my arm was turning blue, beginning the journey I am sharing with you now. That is one of the hardest truths about illness. Sometimes it does not arrive like a single storm that passes through and leaves. Sometimes it begins to braid itself into your life, threading through motherhood, identity, faith, and every plan you thought you had. Sometimes it changes not only your body, but your entire way of living.

That day taught me something I would come to learn again and again: the body speaks, and timing matters. Symptoms are not always small just because they begin quietly. What looks minor at first can become life-threatening very quickly. It was not just the beginning of my illness. It was the beginning of my advocacy."

Struggle

The months that followed were a blur of exhaustion, fear, and logistics. I was a Black woman and a mother with an adult son and a baby girl who depended on me for everything, trying to make sense of a body that no longer felt safe. I cycled through medications and side effects, cried in the shower so no one would hear me, and tried to act stronger than I felt.

Every twinge in my arm felt like a countdown. Every unusual sensation made me wonder if another emergency was coming.

I hated asking for help, but independence was no longer something I could cling to the same way. It had become something I was grieving. That season forced me to face how quickly illness can strip away not only your health, but also your sense of control.

Insight

That first clot taught me that the body speaks, and that timing can decide outcomes.

I realized I had to stop treating symptoms like passing inconveniences and start treating them like information. If I did not pay attention to what I was feeling, when it started, how long it lasted, what made it worse, and what made it better, I would be walking blind into the next emergency. That shift changed me. It made me more observant, more prepared, and more willing to trust what my body was telling me even when other people did not yet understand it. I began to realize that self-advocacy often starts long before the doctor's office. It starts with paying attention.

Guidance

New, severe, or one-sided symptoms should never be brushed aside. This is especially true for pain, swelling, weakness, numbness, or color change. Act first and analyze later.

A few things I wish I had known from the beginning:

- Write symptoms down in the moment if you can. Note the time, location, pain level from 0 to 10, what you were doing, and what made it better or worse.

- If a limb turns blue, turns pale, suddenly swells, becomes weak, or goes numb, seek emergency care right away.
- Have at least two backup people you can call for childcare or transportation in an emergency.
- Keep a simple go-bag ready with your medication list, ID, insurance card, phone charger, and a change of clothes for both you and your child if needed.

I learned these lessons through fear. My prayer is that maybe you will learn them through wisdom instead.

CHAPTER 2

The Diagnosis Journey

The road to diagnosis has been long, frustrating, and exhausting. It was not a straight road, and it was never one of those stories where a person gets sick, sees the right doctor, gets the right test, and walks away with clear answers. My journey was marked by waiting, documenting, asking, researching, and repeating myself. It was shaped by dismissals, dead ends, and the painful gap between what I knew I was feeling and what medicine had not yet figured out how to explain. More often than not, diagnosis came in layers, not all at once.

My story has been one of pushing, waiting, documenting, asking, researching, and repeating myself. It has been a story of being dismissed, trying again, and often living in the painful space between what I knew I was feeling and what medicine had not yet figured out how to explain.

There were times when no one believed me. There were times when my symptoms were brushed aside. There were times when I could see doubt in the room before a word was even spoken. And still, I kept pushing. I had learned something the hard way: when your body keeps sounding an alarm, you cannot afford to stay silent just because someone else does not hear it yet.

More often than not, it took months or even years to get a diagnosis. And the truth is, even now, I am still on that journey.

That is one of the hardest parts for people to understand. They often think diagnosis is a single event, a finish line, or a moment of clarity that settles everything. But for many people living with chronic illness, diagnosis comes in layers. Sometimes one answer opens the door to three more questions. Sometimes you finally get a name for one problem only to realize there are still other things happening that remain unexplained. Sometimes the journey is not toward one diagnosis, but toward many.

That has been my reality. There were tests after tests after tests. There was bloodwork, scans, specialists, procedures, repeat labs, and new consults. There were referrals stacked on top of referrals. Sometimes those tests gave us answers. Sometimes they gave us nothing. And sometimes they gave us just enough information to know that something was wrong, but not enough to tell us exactly why.

That kind of uncertainty is its own kind of exhaustion. It wears on you to keep showing up, keep giving blood, and keep sitting in waiting rooms. You keep hoping this test will finally be the one that explains what is happening, only to leave with another "we're not sure," another "let's keep watching," or another "we may need to send you to someone else."

Early in my journey, I realized I needed to document everything. I tracked what the pain felt like, where it showed up, when it started, and what made it worse or better. I noted patterns in my sleep, food, energy, and ability to function. I took photos of swelling, bruising, skin changes, and anything that might be gone by the time I reached a doctor. That documentation became one of the most powerful tools I had. It helped me see patterns, remember details, and present my case with something stronger than vague memory.

I took photos. I tracked swelling, bruising, skin changes, lumps, and reactions. I tracked the things I knew would be harder to prove if they were gone by the time I got in front of a doctor. I wrote down how I felt emotionally too, because chronic illness affects more than the body. Fear, fatigue, stress, grief, and frustration all become part of the story, and I wanted the full picture in front of me.

That documentation became one of the most powerful tools I had. It helped me see patterns. It helped me remember details when appointments blurred together. And it helped me present my case with something stronger than vague memory.

I showed up to appointments prepared. I brought notes, questions, dates, and details, because I had learned that if I did not protect my own story, it could easily get flattened into one more rushed chart note.

So I made them hear me. I did not do it because I enjoyed pushing or because I wanted conflict. I did it because too much was at stake for me to sit quietly and hope someone else would connect the dots on their own. Through research and documentation, I was actually able to help my doctors diagnose several things. That still says a lot to me. It says that lived experience matters. It says that patients who pay attention can become critical partners in their own care. And it says that sometimes the person living in the body sees the pattern before the medical system does.

At one point, my primary care doctor, Dr. Schlair, submitted my case to the Harvard Undiagnosed Diseases Network. That alone says so much about how medically complex my journey has been. I was not dealing with one simple, easily explained issue. I was living in a body that kept doing things that did not fit neatly into expected categories, and at times even experienced doctors could not fully make sense of it.

I remember how one of my diagnoses came from what seemed like such a simple incident. Right before COVID, I woke up with a stomachache that just would not go away. Of course, I contacted Dr. Schlair, and she told me to come in for a sick visit. She was not in that day, so I saw another doctor instead. They tested my urine and found that my protein level was through the roof.

That led to more testing, then the diagnosis of Chronic Kidney Disease, and then the biopsy. From there came results we had not expected: FSGS. After that, the decision was made to do genetic testing to see whether it had a hereditary cause. The results came back showing Alport Syndrome.

I remember feeling my head spin. It was one more diagnosis, one more thing to process, and one more thing to worry about. I was diagnosed with Alport Syndrome, which is a rare genetic disorder involving abnormal type IV collagen and is often connected to kidney disease, hearing loss, high blood pressure, and eye abnormalities. That diagnosis meant new medications, new side effects, and another layer of concern added to an already complicated life.

In some ways, this diagnosis came more straightforwardly than others. But most of my diagnoses were not that simple. And while I could give you a long list of everything I have been diagnosed with, that is not really the point. I do not want to focus only on the names. I want you to understand the journey, the waiting, the fear, the testing, the uncertainty, and what it costs to keep living through it.

There was a point when we thought we had finally figured out why I kept clotting. For a while, it felt like maybe we were getting somewhere. Maybe this was the answer. Maybe this was the explanation that would finally tie things together. But that turned out to be a dead end.

That is another heartbreak of the diagnosis journey. Sometimes what looks like an answer is only a possibility that later falls apart. And when that happens, you do not just lose information. You lose emotional ground. You lose the hope you had briefly allowed yourself to feel. You have to regroup and begin again.

My hematologist kept searching. Every few months, whenever a new test became available, she would revisit the search. She hoped that maybe this time something would finally point us in the right direction. Maybe this time there would be a marker, a clue, or a result that gave us the answer we had been waiting for. That kind of persistence meant a great deal to me. Even when the answers did not come, it mattered that someone was still looking, still asking questions, and still refusing to give up on finding them.

To this day, my care team is extensive. My team includes primary care, cardiology, rheumatology, neurology, endocrinology, nephrology, gastroenterology, orthopedics, ENT, infectious disease, physical medicine, pain management, orthopedic surgery, ophthalmology, sleep medicine, allergy and immunology, hand surgery, and dermatology.

That is not a health journey. That is an ecosystem. And the fact that it takes that many specialties to manage one life says everything about how layered and complicated chronic illness can become. Every specialist sees one piece of the body or one piece of the puzzle. Part of the burden of being a chronically ill patient is that you often become the bridge between all of them. You are the one carrying the full story from office to office and test to test, trying to make sure the whole picture does not get lost in the fragments.

I am what you call a "super clotter." Even writing those words feels heavy, because it points to one of the most dangerous realities of my health journey. Because of that, I have to stay on blood thinners. And even while on blood thinners, I have still clotted. That fact alone tells you how aggressive and stubborn my condition has been. It is one thing to need medication; it is another thing to still have dangerous events happen while already being treated.

That reality has required constant vigilance, constant adjustment, and constant attention. At this point, I am taking sixteen different medications every single day. Sixteen. That is not a small thing. It is not just swallowing pills. It is managing side effects, timing, interactions, refills, follow-ups, bloodwork, and the emotional reality of living a life that depends on that much medical intervention just to keep functioning and stay safe. Every medication tells part of the story. Every bottle is a reminder that survival has become structured, measured, monitored, and maintained.

And still, I keep going.

That is what I want people to understand about the diagnosis journey. It is not just about finally getting a name. It is about endurance. It is about continuing to show up for yourself while living inside uncertainty. It is about learning how to hold both gratitude for the answers you do get and grief for the ones that still have not come. It is about becoming your own historian, your own witness, and your own advocate. If you do not keep telling the truth of what your body is doing, it can too easily disappear inside a system that prefers simple stories.

My diagnosis journey taught me patience, but not passive patience. It taught me active patience: the kind that keeps records, the kind that asks again, the kind that seeks another opinion, and the kind that keeps researching. It is the kind that allows rest but refuses resignation. It is the kind that understands that "no answer" does not always mean "no problem." Sometimes it just means the right person, the right test, or the right moment has not come yet.

And if you are in that kind of season now, I want you to know something. An unfinished diagnosis journey is still a real journey. You are not less sick because the answers are incomplete. You are not imagining things because the tests do not yet explain everything. You are not dramatic because it has taken years. Sometimes complex bodies require complex searching, and sometimes survival means learning how to keep going while the search continues.

Struggle

The diagnosis journey was exhausting because it demanded so much without always giving clarity in return. I had to keep showing up, keep testing, keep explaining, keep documenting, and keep hoping while often getting only partial answers or none at all. Being dismissed made it heavier. Dead ends made it harder. Living in the space between symptoms and explanation tested my patience, my faith, and my emotional strength. One of the hardest parts was not just the physical suffering; it was living with uncertainty for so long.

Insight

I learned that documentation is power. When answers do not come quickly, details matter. Patterns matter, photos matter, time stamps matter, symptoms matter, and research matters. The more clearly I could tell the story of what my body was doing, the harder it became for my experience to be ignored. I also learned that diagnosis is not always a single moment. Sometimes it is a long unfolding.

Lesson

A delayed diagnosis does not mean your suffering is less real. Keep documenting, keep asking, and keep pushing. An unanswered question is not the same thing as an imaginary problem.

Guidance

A few things that helped me through the diagnosis journey:

- Document everything: symptoms, time of onset, triggers, sleep, food, emotional state, visible changes, medications, and side effects.

- Take photos of anything visible that may change before your appointment.
- Bring a written agenda and timeline to specialist visits so the key facts are clear.
- Keep copies of important labs, scans, reports, and consult notes in one place.
- Ask each specialist: "What are you ruling in?" "What are you ruling out?" "What happens if this test is negative?"
- If one path becomes a dead end, let yourself grieve it, then keep going.
- Sometimes the answer comes slowly. That does not mean you stop searching.

CHAPTER 3

The Revolving Door of Care

After my first clot and the emergency surgery that followed, I was thrust into a new and unfamiliar world. It was the endless revolving door of doctors, specialists, tests, scans, referrals, and follow-up appointments. One appointment led to another referral. One referral led to another waiting room. One waiting room led to another doctor asking me to tell my story from the beginning.

Over and over again, I would repeat my history. Each time I hoped that this doctor would be the one to listen, the one to take me seriously, and the one to help connect the dots. But too often, it felt like I was just another number or another chart. I was another patient moving through a system that had no room for slowness, complexity, or the emotional toll of chronic illness.

Most of the appointments were rushed. Some were dismissive. And for someone like me, living inside a body that seemed to be breaking down in ways no one fully understood, those dismissals were not just frustrating. They were dangerous. I began to realize that if I did not speak up for myself, I would get lost in the shuffle.

I decided to get a second opinion at another hospital just to have another set of eyes on what had become an uncertain and frustrating journey. When I arrived, the vascular surgeon listened carefully as I explained everything that had been happening. After hearing my history, he decided to check the blood pressure in both of my arms. My right arm was fine, but the pressure in my left arm was low, which led him to conclude that I had a partial occlusion.

He immediately called Dr. Patel and explained his findings. This all happened on a Friday, and because it was only a partial occlusion, we believed we had a little time, maybe a few days to a week, before we needed to act. My vascular team advised me to come into the emergency room on Monday so we could deal with it then. They asked if I was comfortable waiting, and I agreed. At the time, I was completely on board with that plan.

But that was not to be.

By Saturday evening, the partial occlusion had become a full-blown clot, and my arm was beginning to turn blue again. Thank God Dr. Patel had given me his cell phone number just in case. A little after 10:00 that Saturday night, I called him to let him know what was happening, and he told me he would meet me at the hospital. When I arrived, he was already waiting outside and rushed me in. I will never forget that.

The doctor at the other hospital who caught the partial occlusion had been sweet, thoughtful, and considerate from the very beginning. I was deeply grateful for the care he showed me. He later told me he was glad I had come to him for the second opinion, but he also explained that my case was very complicated. He encouraged me to stay with the vascular team I already had because it was a strong team. He asked me to call and let him know what happened, and that simple act of care stayed with me.

I can still remember one appointment vividly. I had prepared myself carefully with my notes in hand, my questions written down, and my symptoms tracked. I wanted to make the most of those fifteen minutes because I knew how quickly they would pass. But as soon as I began to talk, the doctor interrupted me.

"Hang on a sec," he said, holding up his hand.

Then he turned back to his computer, typing furiously, scrolling through labs, and clicking through old notes. I waited for him to come back to me, but he never really did. When I tried again, the same thing happened. I was cut off mid-sentence and brushed aside as though what I was experiencing could wait until he was ready to acknowledge it.

The third time he did it, something in me snapped. I stopped him and said firmly, "Before you go any further, I need you to listen to what I have to say. Then we can move forward."

There was a pause. He looked at me, startled, as if no patient had ever demanded his attention so directly. Then he nodded, sat back in his chair, and said quietly, "You're right. I'm sorry. Please, go ahead."

At that moment, I felt a shift. I realized that sometimes you have to claim space for yourself in that tiny exam room. You have to remind them that this is your body, your life, and your pain, not just another chart to update. That appointment taught me something important: advocacy is not always loud or dramatic. Sometimes it is as simple as stopping a doctor in his tracks and insisting on being heard.

And the revolving door did not slow down. There was always another appointment, always another symptom, and always another reason to monitor, document, and decide whether something was serious enough to call about.

I remember one morning waking up with pain in my left hand. I could barely move it. But instead of contacting my doctor right away, I did what I had learned to do so often: I went into monitoring mode. I watched it. I waited. I tried to make sense of it. When you live with chronic illness long enough, that becomes second nature. You are always evaluating.

You are always trying to decide whether this is something temporary, something manageable, or something that needs immediate attention.

After a day or two, the pain still had not gone away, so I messaged Dr. Schlair. As always, she took it seriously and arranged for me to get it checked out, including an ultrasound. When I went in for the ultrasound, I noticed the technician kept going back to the same spot in the palm of my hand. She was quiet in that way medical professionals sometimes get when they are trying not to say too much too soon. Eventually, she called in the doctor.

He looked at the screen, studied it, and then confirmed what none of us expected. I had developed a blood clot in the palm of my hand. Even writing that now still feels surreal. A clot in the palm of my hand. The doctor was kind and caring, but even he was visibly shocked by what he had found. He kept staring at the monitor, almost talking to himself, and finally said, "Is that really a clot? Wow. Haven't seen that before."

That moment stayed with me. It was not because I wanted to impress anyone medically, but because it was one more reminder that my body kept finding new ways to surprise even experienced doctors. It was one more moment of watching a medical professional see something unusual in me and realizing that what I was living with did not fit neatly inside the boxes medicine seemed to prefer.

And that was just another day in the life of a super clotter.

I remember another terrifying moment after a clot removal when I was recovering in the ICU. Suddenly, I saw doctors and nurses rushing into my room. Within moments, I was being raced through the halls while voices shouted to grab the elevator. I was rushed for a CT scan, and that was when they discovered that I was bleeding into my belly. It was one of the scariest moments of my life, and I needed yet another blood transfusion.

The whole scene felt like something out of a television drama, except this was my life and my body on the line. I went back to the ICU for a few more days before eventually being moved to the regular floor and later released. Had those doctors and nurses not been monitoring every blood test so closely and noticed that my blood count was dropping rapidly, I truly do not think I would be here today. That day, they were my heroes.

Another time, I woke up with large red bruises on my body that were so painful all I could do was sit and cry. There were about four of them. The pain was excruciating. It was not the kind of discomfort you can breathe through and keep moving. It was the kind that stops you in your tracks and makes you feel afraid of your own skin. I called for a sick visit with my dermatologist and was in his office within a couple of hours.

To this day, we never fully figured out what was causing them, but he responded quickly and tried to manage what he could. He increased the prednisone I was already taking for something else and added a few other medications to create a kind of cocktail meant to suppress whatever was happening. That is another part of the revolving door people do not always understand. Sometimes you get answers. Sometimes you get management. Sometimes you get a treatment plan without a full explanation. Sometimes the best medicine can offer in that moment is, "Let's try to calm this down."

When your life is medically complicated, that becomes part of the story too. Not every chapter ends with clarity. Some end with partial relief and more unanswered questions. The toll of retelling your story to so many clinicians can be overwhelming. There is something draining about telling the same painful history again and again, only to wait and see whether the person in front of you will really hear it or reduce it to shorthand.

You start to feel like your life has been broken into bullet points: blood clots, stroke, pain, medications, fatigue, procedures, autoimmune disease, kidney disease, Thoracic Outlet Syndrome, fibromyalgia, sleep apnea, side effects, specialists, and follow-ups. At some point, you stop feeling like a person and start feeling like a summary.

And yet, it is still a story worth telling. Because every time I told it clearly, I was creating another opportunity for someone to catch what the last person missed. Every time I spoke up, I was protecting myself from disappearing inside a rushed system. Every time I kept going back, I was choosing not to give up on myself.

But the truth is, sometimes I did want to disappear. Sometimes I wanted to go somewhere quiet and stop explaining. I wanted to stop repeating, stop answering questions, and stop thinking about what my body was doing next.

Sometimes solitude felt easier than advocacy.

But how do you do that when you have children to care for? How do you step away from the world when motherhood still needs you? That became one of the deepest tensions of my life. How do you navigate motherhood and chronic illness at the same time?

The answer is: very carefully.

It is a delicate balancing act, and one that many women struggle with because we are so often taught to prioritize everyone else first. We do what needs to be done. We keep moving. We care for others and push our own needs down the list. But chronic illness forces a different truth. You cannot keep pouring from a body and spirit that are already empty.

We do not get to stop being mothers, but we can learn to care for ourselves in ways that help us continue caring for the people we love. That kind of self-care is not selfish. It is necessary. Sometimes it looks like allowing other people to fill in the gaps, taking your medication the way you should, asking for support, saying no, resting, or letting yourself be helped instead of pretending you are fine. That is the kind of self-care chronic illness taught me. It was not bubble baths and pretty slogans; it was survival care. It was the kind that helps you stay standing long enough to keep loving your family well.

The revolving door of care never really ended. Chronic illness means constant follow-up, new specialists, new symptoms, new questions, and new versions of old fears. But I learned how to walk into each room differently. My questions were written down, my symptoms were tracked, my courage was steadier, and my voice was more practiced. Most importantly, I learned that my time matters too.

My life is not an interruption to someone else's schedule. My pain is not a sidebar. And my story deserves to be told fully, even when the system only wants the short version.

Struggle

Being interrupted, dismissed, and repeatedly forced to retell my story chipped away at my confidence. I dreaded appointments, rehearsed my symptoms in advance, and still often walked out feeling unseen. The power imbalance of white coats versus paper gowns is real. I felt small, rushed, and sometimes reduced to a list of conditions instead of being treated like a whole person. Trying to navigate all of that while also being a mother made it even harder. I was constantly balancing my own medical needs against the emotional and practical needs of my children.

Insight

I learned that I had to bring a blueprint into every visit. If I did not lead with my most urgent concern, the clock would run out before we ever got there. I also learned that repeated telling is not meaningless. Even though it is exhausting, sometimes the story has to be told again because the next person might finally hear what the last one missed. And I learned that self-care in chronic illness is not indulgence; it is part of survival.

Lesson

Lead with your headline: "The most important thing I need to discuss today is because ." Then stop talking until it is acknowledged. And remember: caring for yourself is not taking away from the people you love. It is one of the ways you remain able to love them well.

Guidance

A few things that helped me move through the revolving door of care:

- Prepare a one-to-three item agenda and bring it into every appointment.
- Lead with the most urgent concern first instead of saving it for the end.
- Use respectful interruptions when needed: "I need to finish my thought before we move on."
- Track unusual symptoms carefully, even the ones that sound strange or rare.
- Ask for imaging or follow-up testing when something feels truly wrong.
- Practice survival-focused self-care: rest, medication adherence, support, boundaries, and sleep routines where possible.
- Remember that motherhood does not require you to destroy yourself. Let people fill in the gaps when needed.

You deserve care that sees the whole of you, not just the most convenient part

CHAPTER 4

The Nodule No One Believed

There are moments in this journey that have stayed with me, not only because of the pain itself, but because of the way I was treated when I went looking for help. Some experiences leave a mark on your body. Others leave a mark on your spirit. This was one of those moments.

At that point in my health journey, I had already been through enough to know what it felt like when something in my body was not right. I had learned to pay attention. I had learned not to dismiss strange symptoms just because they seemed hard to explain. My body had already taught me that danger does not always announce itself in obvious ways. Sometimes it arrives quietly. Sometimes it feels strange, vague, or difficult to describe, but that does not make it any less real.

Around that time, I had been waking up regularly with what felt like deep bruises on my body, as if I had been in a fight overnight and somehow missed it. Some of the marks showed on the surface of my skin. They were red, black and blue, or swollen in a way that was impossible to ignore. Other times, it was not a visible bruise so much as a painful lump beneath the surface. On good days I would wake up with a few, but on a bad day it would be more like five to six all over my body. They were tender, sore, and unsettling. It was the kind of pain that made me pause and ask myself, *What now?*

One particular spot on my back concerned me more than the others. It was painful enough that I could not stop thinking about it. Because it was in a place I could not properly examine myself, I asked my son to check it for me. I trusted him to tell me the truth, not what he thought I wanted to hear. When he touched the area, he confirmed exactly what I had been feeling. There was a lump there.

That mattered to me. It was not because I needed someone else to "prove" my pain for it to count, but because it was one more confirmation that I was not imagining what I felt in my own body. I knew something was there, and now someone else could feel it too.

So I made an appointment with my then primary care doctor. I went in expecting concern, or at the very least a proper examination. I explained what had been happening. I told her about the painful bruised feeling, the swelling, and the lump on my back. I told her how alarming it was to keep waking up with new areas of pain and unexplained changes in my body. I was not asking for drama. I was asking for care. I was asking her to take a closer look.

Instead, she lightly brushed her hand across my back and said flatly, "I don't feel anything."

That alone would have been upsetting enough. But before I could even fully process her dismissal, she added, "Maybe you should see a therapist."

Her words hit me like a punch in the chest. It was not because I have anything against therapy. In fact, I was already seeing a therapist to help me carry the emotional and mental weight of everything I had been going through. She knew that. She knew my history. She knew how serious my medical journey had already been. She knew the trauma, the fear, the uncertainty, and the emotional toll of living in a body that had already betrayed me in terrifying ways.

And still, instead of examining me properly, she chose to suggest that this pain was somehow in my head. I was stunned. There are some moments when disbelief leaves you speechless, and there are other moments when it lights a fire in you. For me, it did both.

I looked at her and said, "You've been my doctor since the beginning. You've seen what I've gone through. How dare you tell me that this is in my head without even examining me properly?"

She repeated herself: "I just don't feel anything."

That was it. There was no deeper examination and no curiosity. There were no follow-up questions and no attempt to investigate further. There was no acknowledgment of my history, my fear, my pain, or the simple possibility that maybe, just maybe, I knew what I was talking about.

I left that office angry, humiliated, and hurt. There is a particular kind of pain that comes from being dismissed by someone who has known your story. It is bad enough when a stranger doubts you. It cuts deeper when the doubt comes from someone who has already seen what you have survived. It was someone who should know better. It was someone who should at least know that you are not casually inventing lumps and pain for attention.

As I walked out of that office, I replayed the appointment in my mind. Did I explain it badly? Did I sound too emotional? Did I not say enough? Was I overreacting?

That is the cruelty of medical dismissal. It does not just deny your experience in the moment. It can follow you home and make you question yourself long after the appointment is over. It can make you replay your own reality like a bad recording, wondering if maybe you somehow got it wrong. That kind of doubt is dangerous. Because when people are made to question themselves often enough, they start staying quiet about things they should absolutely speak up about.

A day later, I went to a physical therapy session. I did not walk in expecting some dramatic turning point. It was just the next thing on the schedule. But during the session, I mentioned the pain in my back and the lump I had tried to get my doctor to examine. My therapist stopped what he was doing and came over to check the area.

This time, someone actually looked. This time, someone actually examined me. The moment his hand pressed against my back, he froze.

"I feel it," he said quietly. "There's definitely a nodule here. I don't know what it is, but I think we need to cancel all sessions until you have this checked out further."

I cannot fully describe the relief I felt in that moment. It was not relief because the problem was solved; it wasn't. It was not relief because I suddenly had answers; I didn't. It was relief because I had been validated. Someone else felt it. Someone else saw what my doctor had chosen not to see. Someone else confirmed that I was not imagining it, not exaggerating, and not creating symptoms out of fear or stress. There was something there. I had known it, and now someone else knew it too.

That moment mattered more than it may seem on the surface. Because with chronic illness, validation is not a small thing. When your reality has been doubted often enough, being believed can feel like oxygen. It can steady you. It can pull you back from that frightening edge where self-doubt starts replacing self-trust.

That experience cemented one of the hardest lessons of my journey: not every doctor will believe you. And when they don't, it is not only okay to walk away. It is necessary.

I decided to file a formal complaint against that primary care doctor. That decision was not about revenge. It was not about wanting to embarrass her, punish her, or "get even." It was about accountability. It was about naming what had happened and refusing to normalize it. It was about making sure there was at least some record that this kind of dismissal had occurred. And it was about protecting the next patient. It was for the one who might be more fragile or more easily silenced, the one who might hear "Maybe you should see a therapist" and go home believing her own pain did not deserve another look.

I could not let that be the end of the story. So I also made another decision: I found a new primary care provider.

That choice was not easy. Starting over with a new doctor can feel exhausting. You have to retell your history, rebuild trust, and explain the timeline. You have to hope again and risk disappointment again. There is a temptation to stay with a dismissive provider simply because the process of starting over feels like too much.

But I had learned enough by then to know this: staying with someone who dismisses your pain is more dangerous than the inconvenience of finding someone new. A provider does not have to have every answer. They do not have to be perfect. But they do need to be willing to listen, examine, ask questions, and treat you with dignity. If they are unwilling to do that, they are not a safe place for your care.

That nodule may never have received a neat diagnosis. There was no tidy ending to that part of the story and no dramatic reveal that tied everything up with a bow. But even without a perfect medical conclusion, the experience taught me something far more important.

It taught me that I must trust myself. It taught me that my body's signals are real, even when someone else refuses to honor them. It taught me that dismissal is not the same thing as truth. And it taught me that if one doctor will not listen, I have every right to find one who will.

That lesson has carried me through many moments since then. Chronic illness will test more than your body. It will test your confidence, your patience, and your trust in yourself. It will put you in rooms where you have to decide whether you believe your own lived experience enough to keep pushing when someone with credentials is telling you to sit down and be quiet.

Sometimes it simply means you are standing in front of the wrong person. And when that happens, walking away is not weakness. It is wisdom.

Struggle

Not being believed made me question my own body in ways that were deeply unsettling. I replayed that visit over and over, wondering if I had explained badly, sounded too emotional, or somehow made too much of what I was feeling. That is what gaslighting can do. It can make you question your own reality. That kind of doubt is dangerous. It keeps people quiet when they should speak up and keeps people home when they should seek care. For me, the struggle was not only the physical pain of the nodule itself. It was the emotional wound of being treated like my body could not be trusted, even by someone who had been part of my care for years.

Insight

A dismissal is data. It is not data about you; it is data about the provider. When someone will not properly examine you, will not palpate the exact area you are describing, and will not ask thoughtful follow-up questions, that tells you something important about the quality of care you are receiving. It does not mean your symptoms are imaginary. It means you may be standing in front of someone who is unwilling or unable to meet the moment.

Lesson

If your lived experience and the provider's conclusion do not match, and you have not been properly examined, you are allowed to change clinicians. You are allowed to protect yourself from poor care. You are allowed to want better.

Guidance

A few things I learned from this experience:

- Ask for a focused exam: "Can you palpate the exact area while I point to it?"
- Get a second opinion when needed from another doctor, a nurse practitioner, or even a physical therapist who may notice what someone else overlooked.
- Bring written notes and photos of visible changes such as swelling, bruising, or redness.
- Document dismissive statements as closely to word-for-word as possible in your journal.
- If imaging or labs seem reasonable and are refused, ask that the refusal and the reason be documented in your chart.
- Do not stay with a provider who consistently makes you feel small, unheard, or ashamed for reporting symptoms.

Your pain is not less real because someone failed to respect it.

CHAPTER 5

The Doctor Who Listens

Not every doctor in my journey dismissed me. Some, though far too rare, became lifelines. Finding them felt like stumbling across an oasis after wandering through a desert of indifference. After enough rushed appointments, clipped responses, and cold exam rooms where I felt more like a problem than a person, I had almost forgotten what it felt like to sit across from someone in medicine who actually knew how to listen.

Then I met the doctor who would become the most important person on my care team: Dr. Sheira Schlair, an internist.

I still remember that first appointment vividly. She walked into the room, introduced herself, and from the very beginning, something felt different. Before she touched the computer, before she opened the chart, and before she started scanning labs or test results, she sat down. She looked me in the eye and said, "Tell me your story."

That simple invitation changed the whole atmosphere. It may sound small to someone who has never had to fight to be heard, but to me it felt enormous. It told me immediately that I was not just another chart or another diagnosis. I was not just another body being moved through the system. In that moment, I felt that she understood something many providers miss: illness happens to a whole person, not just a body part.

So I told her. I told her about my symptoms, my history, and my clotting. I told her about the surgeries, the fear, and the frustration. I shared the experiences of appointments where I had felt ignored, the weight of trying to mother through crisis, and the exhaustion of carrying both the illness and the burden of proving it over and over again. I expected interruptions because by then I had grown used to them. I expected her attention to drift toward the screen. I expected to feel the pressure of the clock.

But she stayed with me. She listened. She asked thoughtful questions that told me she had not only heard my words but understood their weight. She did not rush me past the parts that mattered. She did not cut me off to chase her own agenda. She did not make me feel like I needed to perform my pain in just the right way to earn her concern.

At the end of that appointment, she pulled her chair a little closer and said, "Here's the plan. We'll take it step by step, and you won't walk this road alone."

I walked out of that office in tears. It was not because I was afraid or because I had gotten devastating news. I cried because I felt seen. When you have spent enough time being dismissed, being seen can feel like a miracle.

That appointment reminded me of something I had almost started to forget: good care is not only about intelligence. It is also about presence. It is about whether a provider has the willingness to slow down long enough to recognize the human being sitting in front of them. It is about whether they understand that fear, uncertainty, and exhaustion are not side notes to illness. They are part of it.

A few months later, I had another appointment with her that stayed with me just as deeply. By then, I had become more organized in how

I approached my care. I came in with my notes, my questions, and my medication concerns. I brought the side effects I had been tracking and changes I had noticed in my bloodwork. I had learned by then that I needed to come prepared, because chronic illness does not leave room for vagueness. You learn to collect details because details can matter. You learn to bring receipts because your body often has to be translated into language other people will respect.

When she saw how prepared I was, she smiled and said, "Good. You came prepared. I have an agenda as well, so let's go through these one by one."

That moment meant more to me than she probably realized. She did not roll her eyes at my notes. She did not treat my preparation as anxiety, overthinking, or an inconvenience. She welcomed it and made space for it. She treated my advocacy as something useful rather than something irritating. In her presence, I did not feel like I had to apologize for caring deeply about my own body. I did not feel like I had to shrink my questions to make myself more comfortable to manage.

She saw my preparation as partnership, and that is what good care feels like. It does not punish you for being informed or make you feel difficult for asking questions. What made her even more special was that her care was not only clinical; it was deeply human.

Sometimes, before we even started going over our agenda, she would pause and ask, "Before we move forward, how are you really doing? Not just physically, but spiritually and emotionally?"

She asked because she knew I was struggling emotionally as well. As a Christian woman, this was a season of questioning for me. It was a season where faith was still present, but so were grief, confusion, and exhaustion. That question always reached deeper than the others.

The truth is that chronic illness never stays neatly in the body. It spills into everything. It touches your mind, your faith, your energy, and your family. It affects your finances, your relationships, your sense of safety, and your identity. It changes how you wake up, how you rest, how you hope, and how you pray. To have a doctor acknowledge that was no small thing. It told me she understood that healing and care are not just about lab numbers or medication adjustments. They are also about the person carrying all of it.

One day, after an especially hard appointment, she ended our visit by asking, "Can I give you a hug?"

Even now, writing those words makes me pause. In a system that can often feel cold, detached, and transactional, that moment of compassion broke through like sunlight. It was a small gesture, but it carried enormous meaning. It reminded me that medicine does not have to lose its humanity to be professional. Compassion is not weakness. Kindness is not fluff. Presence is not extra. For patients carrying long-term pain, fear, and uncertainty, those things can become part of the healing too.

That doctor reminded me that while the healthcare system often fails, individual humanity can still break through the cracks. The contrast between her and some of my other doctors could not have been clearer. Around that same time, I saw another doctor in the same hospital system who barely looked at me at all. He came into the room, glanced at the chart, rattled off instructions, and left in less than five minutes. There were no real questions, no real curiosity, and no effort to understand how I was doing beyond whatever was already written down.

I remember sitting there afterward thinking, *How can two people in the same profession treat patients so differently?*

That question stayed with me. It showed me something I needed to fully understand: the letters behind a person's name do not tell you everything about how they will care for you. Two doctors can have similar training, similar credentials, and similar access to the same hospital system, yet still offer completely different experiences to the human beings in their care. One can leave you feeling dismissed, managed, and rushed. Another can leave you feeling respected, partnered with, and safe.

That realization changed the way I thought about finding care. I stopped thinking of it as luck and started seeing it as courage. It was the courage to keep searching. It was the courage to leave the familiar when the familiar is not serving you. It was the courage to trust your instincts when something feels off and the courage to believe that you deserve better even when the system trains you to settle for less.

For many of us, especially Black women, there is often an unspoken pressure to be "good patients." We feel pressured to be agreeable, to be grateful for whatever we get, and to not seem difficult. We try not to ask too much or challenge the expert in the room. We try not to make waves.

But illness teaches you quickly that loyalty to poor care is not a virtue; it is a risk. There comes a point when staying with the wrong provider is more dangerous than the discomfort of finding a new one.

Finding this doctor took time. It took years, insurance hurdles, disappointment, and dead ends. It took the emotional effort of beginning again after being let down. Switching providers is not simple. It can bring guilt, uncertainty, paperwork, and fatigue. It can make you question whether starting over is worth it.

She reminded me that I was not asking for too much by wanting to be heard. She reminded me that my whole self belonged in the room. That kind of doctor does more than prescribe. She restores dignity, trust, and the sense that you still matter.

I did not need someone who was merely smart. I needed someone who was clinically sharp and emotionally present. I needed someone who understood the medicine and also understood the person carrying the diagnosis. I needed someone who welcomed me as a partner instead of treating me like an inconvenience.

That kind of doctor does more than prescribe. That kind of doctor restores trust. And sometimes, trust is part of what helps the body keep going.

The doctor who listens does not just hear symptoms. She hears fear. She hears fatigue. She hears what is said and sometimes what is not said. He or she understands that patients are not machines presenting malfunctions. They are people trying to live, love, parent, work, and survive. They are trying to hold themselves together while their bodies do uncertain things.

The doctor who listens reminds you that you matter. And sometimes, that can be as healing as any medication.

Struggle

One of the hardest parts of this journey was learning how much damage dismissive care had done to my spirit. By the time I met Dr. Schlair, I had grown so used to being rushed, interrupted, and minimized that I almost expected it. I had learned to brace myself before appointments, to prepare for indifference, and to carry the emotional weight of not knowing whether the person in front of me would actually hear me. That kind of medical fatigue is real. It makes trust difficult, hope fragile, and starting over with a new provider feels exhausting.

Finding a doctor who truly listened was a gift, but it also made me realize how much I had been surviving without. It showed me just how deeply I had been craving care that felt safe, human, and respectful. In that realization, there was both comfort and grief.

Insight

I learned that the right doctor can change more than your treatment plan. They can change how safe you feel in your own care. Being listened to reminded me that I was not asking for too much by wanting compassion, clarity, and partnership. It showed me that good care is not only about credentials or clinical skill. It is also about presence, dignity, and the willingness to truly see the person behind the symptoms.

Lesson

Do not settle for care that makes you feel small. A good doctor does not make you fight to be heard at every visit. A good doctor listens, explains, respects your preparation, and welcomes your voice as part of the process. The right provider may not have every answer right away, but they will not make you feel invisible while searching for them.

Guidance

A few things I learned from finding the right doctor:

- Pay attention to how you feel after the appointment. If you leave feeling dismissed, rushed, confused, or ashamed, that matters.
- A strong provider does not just treat symptoms. They make space for your questions, your fears, and your lived experience.
- Bring your notes, your timeline, and your concerns without apology. The right doctor will see your preparation as partnership rather than a problem.
- If a doctor consistently makes you feel unheard, it is okay to look elsewhere. Starting over can be exhausting, but staying with the wrong provider can cost even more.
- Trust the difference between being managed and being cared for. Your body knows when a space feels safe.

Sometimes healing begins the moment you realize you deserve better care than what you have been receiving.

CHAPTER 6

The Stroke That Changed Everything

There are days that leave marks on your life so deep that everything after them feels different. For me, one of those days was the morning I had a stroke.

I had not been feeling well the day before. It was hard to explain exactly what was wrong, which is often one of the hardest parts of living with chronic illness. Not every warning sign arrives with a clear label. Sometimes your body simply feels off, heavy, drained, and unfamiliar in a way that is impossible to ignore. That is how I felt. I knew something was not right, even though I could not yet name it.

That is how I felt that day. My body was heavy, my energy was low, and I knew something was not right. I tried to keep track of my symptoms in my journal, as I had trained myself to do by then, but I still could not quite explain what felt different. I just knew I did not feel like myself. There was a quiet wrongness in my body. It was the kind of feeling that makes you uneasy even when you cannot neatly describe it.

I remember telling my aide, Stephanie, who had been by my side for a few years at that point, that something was not right. She listened with a calm but concerned expression and told me to let her know if I needed anything. She said she would keep a close eye on me.

There was comfort in that. When you live with chronic illness, you learn the value of people who pay attention, people who do not panic, do not minimize, and understand that when you say something feels off, it matters.

A little after Stephanie had helped me to shower and started breakfast, I stepped out of the bathroom and wrapped myself in a towel. It should have been an ordinary moment. It was one of those simple in-between moments in a day that barely registers in memory. But as I stepped forward, I suddenly felt a strange pulling sensation in my face. It was immediate and unnatural.

I walked toward Stephanie and tried to speak, but my words came out slurred. She looked at me, and I could see fear rise in her eyes.

"Kay, your face!" she said.

I hurried to a mirror with my left side barely moving and saw it. My reflection was twisted and one side of my face was drooping. It is a terrible thing to look into a mirror and see your body doing something you know it should not be doing. It was not subtle, and it was not something I could explain away. I knew instantly what was happening. I was having a stroke.

In that moment, something inside me went completely still. Fear was there, of course, but clarity was stronger. I did not have the luxury of falling apart. I did not have time to second-guess myself, to wait and see, or to call five different people for opinions. I knew what this was, and I knew we had to move.

I told Stephanie we needed to get to the hospital immediately. Within minutes, we were on our way. By the grace of God, we arrived within twenty to thirty minutes of the onset. That timing mattered more than words can fully express.

Because of my history of blood clots and previous mini-strokes, the doctors understood the urgency right away. They did not have to waste precious time figuring out whether this was serious. They already knew I was high-risk, and they moved quickly. In the emergency room, they administered the clot-busting drug tPA.

Then something extraordinary happened. We watched my face begin to return. The droop that had twisted my reflection started to ease. The paralysis that had altered my appearance began to lift. It felt almost as if a tide had turned in real time. Everyone around me seemed amazed at how well I was doing, and I could hear some of the nurses quietly whispering the word "miracle" under their breath.

I remember asking one of them, "Why does everyone keep calling it a miracle?"

She looked at me gently and said, "Because we almost never see patients arrive this quickly. Most people call a family member, wait to see if it passes, or second-guess themselves. In doing that, they lose precious time. By the time they reach us, it is often too late for the tPA to work as it should. But you came straight in without hesitation, and that saved your life."

Her words stayed with me. They still do. She was naming something bigger than just my story. She was naming something so many women live inside of without even realizing it. We are so often trained to minimize our symptoms, push through discomfort, or put everyone else first. We tell ourselves we are probably overreacting. We tell ourselves to rest first, pray first, or see how we feel in an hour.

But a stroke does not wait for convenience. Neither does time.

How many lives are forever changed because people hesitate? How many outcomes are worse because someone waited? How many women have brushed off terrifying symptoms because they were so used to caring for others that they no longer knew how to center their own survival?

That day taught me with brutal clarity that symptoms like sudden facial drooping, slurred speech, weakness, or numbness are not things you negotiate with. You act. You go. You get help. That is it. There is no debate, no delay, and no trying to be polite to your own emergency.

The stroke also deepened my understanding of what it means to live with chronic illness. People often think chronic illness is only about the daily management of symptoms, medications, and appointments. And yes, it is those things, but it is also this: living with the constant knowledge that life can change in an instant. Your body can shift between one breath and the next. An ordinary morning can suddenly become a medical emergency.

That awareness changes you. It changes the way you listen to your body and the way you prepare. It changes the way you move through the world and how you think about time, risk, and survival.

When people say to me now, "You're so strong," I often think back to that day. Strength did not feel glamorous. It looked like survival. It looked like staying calm while fear rose in Stephanie's eyes. It looked like moving while my body was trying to betray me.

That stroke changed more than my medical story. It changed me. Afterward, I became sharper and more vigilant. I paid even closer attention to changes in my face, my speech, and my coordination. I began listening for slurring in my own words. I checked my smile in the mirror. I learned to notice little shifts that other people might not even think about.

The body remembers trauma, and so does the mind. Even after the immediate danger passed, the fear lingered. Recovery was not just physical; it was psychological too. It is one thing to survive a stroke. It is another thing to live after one, carrying the memory of how fast it happened and how different the ending could have been if I had delayed.

I taught my children what to watch for. I made sure the people close to me, including Stephanie, understood the signs. I began to see emergency plans differently, not as something negative, but as something loving and necessary. Preparation is not fear. Preparation is care. It is one of the most practical forms of self-advocacy there is.

The stroke also gave me something I carry with me now whenever I speak about health advocacy: a story that might help save somebody else. If sharing what happened to me helps one person recognize the warning signs in their own body or in someone they love, then this chapter is doing holy work. So much of advocacy begins with awareness.

Sometimes people do not act because they do not know. Sometimes they have never been told just how quickly minutes can become destiny.

I know now, and I want other people to know too. That day reminded me yet again that advocating for my health is not optional. It is not extra. It is not something nice to do if I have the energy. It is life-saving.

The stroke that changed everything also changed the way I understand urgency, preparation, and grace. What happened in that emergency room felt like a miracle, but it was a miracle made possible by action, awareness, and refusing to wait. Sometimes that is how miracles come, not by removing the crisis, but by making a way through it.

Struggle

After the stroke, fear did not disappear just because I survived. It lingered. I listened for slurs in my speech. I traced my smile in the mirror. I paid attention to every strange sensation in my face and every unusual feeling that might have meant something was happening again. I taught my children what to do if it ever returned, and I carried the quiet fear of how quickly life could change.

The body remembers trauma, and so does the mind. Recovery was physical, but it was also emotional and psychological. Surviving the event was one thing; learning how to live after it, without being ruled by fear every second, was something else entirely.

Insight

Preparation is a form of love. Having an emergency plan does not invite disaster; it reduces harm when minutes matter. Knowing where to go, what hospital you prefer, what medications you take, and how to describe your symptoms can make all the difference in a crisis. That stroke taught me that preparation is not pessimism. It is wisdom. It is a way of loving yourself and protecting your future when time is critical.

Lesson

Act FAST for stroke: Face drooping, Arm weakness, Speech difficulty, and Time to call 911. Do not wait to see if it passes. Do not talk yourself out of urgency. Do not drive yourself if it can be avoided. Time matters.

Guidance

A few things I learned that may help someone else:

- Post your emergency plan somewhere visible, like the refrigerator, and teach everyone in your household the steps and key phone numbers.
- Keep an updated one-page medical summary with your diagnoses, medications, allergies, surgeries, and specialist contacts.
- Practice describing symptoms with clear time stamps, such as: "Onset at 8:35 a.m., slurred speech, left facial droop."
- Teach your children or close family members the warning signs of stroke so they know when to act.
- After discharge, schedule a follow-up with your primary care doctor or specialist to review likely causes and prevention steps.

- Never minimize sudden neurological changes. Sudden weakness, facial drooping, numbness, confusion, or slurred speech should always be treated as urgent.

Your quick action can save your life.

CHAPTER 7

Life Between Emergencies

People often pay attention to the emergencies. They understand the ambulance moments, the surgeries, the hospital stays, the strokes, and the blood clots. People often pay attention to the emergencies. They understand the ambulance moments, the surgeries, the hospital stays, the strokes, and the blood clots. Those are the moments that look dramatic from the outside, the moments people can point to and say, "That must have been hard." And they are hard. But what many people do not see is the life that happens between emergencies, the quiet suffering, the daily burden, and the exhausting, unglamorous work of trying to live inside a body that hurts every single day.

Life between emergencies has been rough. There are good days and bad days, and there are days when I feel so worn down that I just want to give up. That is the truth.

Because chronic illness is not only about surviving the big medical events. It is also about surviving the ordinary days that never really feel ordinary anymore. It is about waking up every morning and not knowing exactly which version of your body you are going to get. It is about trying to build a life around unpredictability. It is about functioning, mothering, showing up, and carrying responsibility while pain remains the one constant you can count on.

My daily life consists of doctor's appointments, medications three times a day, and stomach issues from all the medication. It is about trying to manage a body that does not move through the world easily. There are days when I am unsteady on my feet and days when I cannot shower by myself. There are days when I survive on little or no sleep.

There are days when my hands are so swollen that I can barely use them. There are days when I wake up so puffy that I hardly recognize myself. There are days when I am so exhausted I can barely stand, and days when my mind is so foggy that I cannot focus on anything for long. And yet, even in the middle of all of that, there are still days when I push through.

I push through to show up for the people I love, for my community, and for myself. But no matter how I show up, the pain does not go away. That is one of the hardest truths of this life.

Pain has been the main constant in my life for the last fifteen years. I have honestly forgotten what it feels like to live in a body without pain. Pain is not an occasional visitor in my life; it is a daily presence woven into everything. It is something I wake up to, carry through the day, and try to rest around at night.

Sleep, especially, has become its own struggle. Most days I get anywhere from one hour to five hours of sleep. Because I also struggle with sleep apnea, it is never truly good sleep. Sleep is something most people look forward to, but for me, it is something I often dread. There is no safe or comfortable position for me to sleep in. Between the residual effects of the stroke, torn rotator cuffs on both sides, constant back pain, stomach pain, headaches, and fibromyalgia, lying down does not automatically mean rest. It often just means a new angle of pain.

That changes your relationship with night and your relationship with rest. When sleep becomes something you cannot trust, your whole day starts from behind. Waking up exhausted is normal for me. I do not wake up refreshed. I wake up already feeling like I have been fighting before the day has even started.

Once I am up, it becomes about one thing: surviving the day. I know that may sound dramatic to some people, but for me it is not dramatic. It is honest. On many days, that really is my only job.

Most days I wake up swollen from head to toe, sometimes with bruises, and always feeling worse for wear. Then comes the routine of taking the many medications I need just to stay on my feet. Some of these medications I have been taking for years, and you would think that over time my body would adjust and the side effects would ease up. But that has not always been the case. With some of them, the side effects still hit me as if I were taking them for the very first time. My body never fully adjusted, so I still feel it all.

I feel the stomach aches, the diarrhea, the dizziness, the sleepiness, the nausea, and the blurred vision. If I take my medications at 8:00 in the morning, I may be of no use to myself until three or four in the afternoon. There are some days when I simply cannot function at all.

That is another part of life between emergencies people do not understand. Sometimes the treatment becomes its own burden. Sometimes the medicine that is helping keep you alive also takes so much out of you that the day feels half lost before it even begins. You do not just manage illness; you manage the fallout of managing illness.

That kind of life requires help. There are times when I need help getting out of bed. Most days I need help showering and getting dressed. There are times when my food has to be completely cut up because my hands are not strong enough to do it myself. There are days when basic tasks become team efforts. There are days when the woman other people see is not the woman who needed help just to get ready that morning.

One of the hardest parts of all of this has been depending on my son to help take care of me. That has been one of my deepest struggles over the years. Losing my independence has been one of the hardest things to accept in this life. There is grief in needing help. There is grief in once being able to do simple things for yourself and then having to ask someone else to step in. There is grief in feeling like the role is backwards, in watching your child take care of you in ways you never imagined he would have to. Even when that care is given with love, it can still ache. Love does not erase the grief; it just helps carry it.

The job of staying alive is overwhelming on so many levels. It is not only about getting through the obvious big things. It is also about being hyper-focused on the smallest things. I am watching my body, my symptoms, and my side effects. I am paying attention to swelling, bruising, pain levels, dizziness, diet, timing, hydration, sleep, medication reactions, and all the tiny shifts that might mean something bigger is brewing underneath the surface.

That kind of vigilance is exhausting. It is a full-time mental job even when it is invisible to everyone else. And one of the most frustrating parts is that I do not look like I am at death's door. People will say, "But you don't look sick." My honest question is: how am I supposed to look?

People seem to think that being chronically ill means you should always look worn down, broken, and terrible. But I refuse to fit inside that box. I refuse to look like what my body feels like.

So yes, I fake it. Yes, I do. I push through the pain, the exhaustion, the side effects, and the fear. I move with purpose because I cannot afford not to. When people see me smiling, dressed, speaking, or showing up with joy, I need them to understand that it does not mean the pain is gone. It does not always mean it is a good day. It often just means I do not want you to see behind the facade. It means I do not want pity. It means I am choosing dignity in the middle of suffering.

That is one of the quiet complexities of chronic illness. Sometimes surviving looks polished from the outside. Sometimes strength wears lipstick. Sometimes endurance shows up smiling. People mistake presentation for ease, but ease is not what is happening. Work is what is happening. Effort is what is happening. Courage is what is happening.

Life between emergencies has taught me a different kind of courage than the emergency room ever could. Emergency courage is fast. It is adrenaline. It is urgency. It is action in a crisis. But the courage of daily life is slower. It is quieter. It is waking up to the same pain and choosing not to surrender to it. It is facing the same limitations and still trying to find meaning inside them. It is accepting help without letting it strip you of dignity. It is learning how to live a life that may not look like the one you planned, while still refusing to call it over.

That is the work of the in-between. And sometimes, the in-between is where the deepest resilience is built. This life has taught me that survival is not found only in the dramatic moments. Sometimes it looks like taking your medicine or asking for help. Sometimes it looks like letting your son cut your food when your hands cannot do it. Sometimes it looks like resting without guilt or making it through one more day in a body that hurts. And that matters too.

If you are reading this and living a life between emergencies, I want you to know that the ordinary suffering counts. The daily struggle counts. The things no one claps for, the things no one sees, and the things you quietly carry just to get through a day count.

And so do you.

Struggle

The hardest part of life between emergencies is that the pain never fully leaves. There is no real break from it. It follows me into the ordinary parts of life and makes simple things hard. Bathing, walking, eating, sleeping, standing, focusing, and even resting are not automatic for me. They are daily challenges. On top of that, medication side effects, swelling, bruising, exhaustion, sleep deprivation, stomach issues, and brain fog create another layer of difficulty. Some days I do not recognize myself physically. Other days I cannot think clearly enough to function well. There are days when simply staying alive feels like the job.

Insight

I learned that surviving the in-between requires as much strength as surviving the emergency. The world often sees the dramatic moments, but chronic illness is also built out of quiet battles. It is built of daily pain, daily management, and daily adaptation. The ordinary days are not easy just because they are not emergencies. In many ways, they require a deeper and steadier kind of resilience. I also learned that presentation is not the same as wellness. Looking okay does not mean I am okay.

Lesson

Life between emergencies is still real illness. Just because the crisis is not visible does not mean the suffering is gone. The in-between matters.

Guidance

A few things that help me navigate the daily reality of chronic illness:

- Create routines for medications, meals, appointments, and rest as much as your body allows.
- Ask for help with practical tasks like shopping, cooking, cleaning, dressing, bathing, and transportation.
- Pay attention to side effects and document them, especially if they interfere with your daily functioning.

- Give yourself permission to rest without feeling like you have failed.
- Do not measure your worth by how much you can physically do in a day.
- Be honest with at least a few trusted people about what your "good" and "bad" days really look like.
- Remember that smiling and showing up do not erase what your body is carrying.
- Sometimes making it through the day is enough, and sometimes that is a victory all by itself.

CHAPTER 8

Learning to Speak the Language

When I first entered the world of chronic illness, I felt like a stranger in a foreign country. The doctors spoke in acronyms and shorthand, using words I could barely pronounce and much less understand. I would sit there nodding politely and trying not to look confused. I tried not to interrupt and tried to keep up with conversations that were supposed to be about my own body but somehow felt like they were happening around me instead of with me.

At first, I left appointments more confused than when I arrived. I would sit in the car afterward and stare at my notes, frustrated and overwhelmed, looking at lab names, medication names, and terminology I did not understand. I felt the weight of how dangerous that confusion really was. How could I make decisions about my health if I did not even understand what was being said?

That question changed everything for me. I realized that if I wanted to be taken seriously and if I wanted to stay alive, I had to learn the language of medicine. It did not happen overnight. I did not wake up one day suddenly confident and fluent in medical terminology. It came little by little, the way most real learning does.

I started small. Whenever I heard a term I did not understand, I wrote it down. When I got home, I looked it up. I kept a running list in my journal of unfamiliar words and what they meant. I tracked words like thrombosis, subclavian, embolism, aneurysm, etiology, differential diagnosis, and INR. At first they sounded intimidating, but the more I learned, the less power they had to make me feel small.

I learned that INR stood for International Normalized Ratio, which is a measure of how thin or thick my blood was while I was taking anticoagulants. I learned that etiology meant the cause of a condition. I learned that differential diagnosis meant the list of possible explanations a doctor is considering before settling on one. I learned what terms meant on my scans, in my labs, and in my chart.

That knowledge gave me something precious: confidence. It was not arrogance or the illusion that I knew more than my doctors. It was simply confidence. It was the kind that comes when confusion no longer owns the room.

The next time I sat in an appointment and a doctor rattled off technical language, I did not just nod automatically. I stopped them and said, "Can you explain what that means for me in plain English?"

I will never forget the look on one doctor's face the first time I said that. At first he seemed surprised. Then he smiled and said, "Absolutely. Thank you for asking." He broke it down in a way I could actually carry with me. That moment may have seemed small to him, but it mattered to me. It taught me that asking for clarity was not rude; it was responsible. It was not a sign that I was not smart enough. It was a sign that I was engaged enough to want to understand.

Understanding matters. If you do not understand, you cannot truly consent, weigh your options, or fully participate in your own care.

Learning the language also helped me catch mistakes. There was a time when a nurse told me that my INR was "stable" when in fact it was dangerously high. If I had still been the woman I was at the beginning of this journey, I might have nodded and gone home. But by that point, I knew what those numbers meant. I knew enough to ask questions and say, "That does not sound right." That questioning led to changes in my medication that likely prevented another clot.

That mattered. When you live with chronic illness, knowledge is not just empowering in some abstract way. Sometimes it is protective. Sometimes it is the thing standing between you and harm.

I also remember appointments where learning the language changed the whole tone of the room. When I started using the right words for what I was experiencing, some doctors listened differently. When I could describe symptoms more precisely and connect them to previous diagnoses, the conversation shifted. I stopped feeling like I was begging to be understood and started feeling like an actual participant in my care.

I could say things like, "I'm concerned about the clotting risk," or "This side effect is interfering with my ability to function." I could ask if a symptom fit the differential diagnosis they were considering or ask for the rationale behind a treatment. That kind of language did not make me less human; it made me less helpless. There is a difference.

I want to be clear about something: learning the language was never about becoming cold or purely clinical. It was not about turning myself into a walking chart or stripping emotion out of the room. It was about making sure emotion was not the only thing I had to rely on when the room started moving too fast.

Pain can make your thoughts cloudy. Fear can make it hard to remember what was said. Fatigue can make everything blur together. If all you leave with is emotion, you may forget the actual information you need.

That is why I began writing everything down. I recorded terminology, medication names, test names, lab results, questions, and definitions. Over time, that journal became part glossary, part survival guide. It became a bridge between what was happening in the room and what I could understand afterward. The more I learned, the less afraid I was to say, "Hold on. Can you say that another way?"

That sentence became one of the most powerful tools I had. It was honest, clear, and refused to let pride or intimidation get in the way of my understanding. That was another lesson I had to learn: pride has no place in a medical crisis. If you do not understand, ask. If you forget, ask again. If the explanation still does not make sense, ask for another version. Your health is too important to leave the room confused just because you do not want to look uninformed.

Over time, I became fluent enough to advocate more effectively. Doctors began to see me as a partner. They noticed the way I came prepared and the way I asked questions. They noticed the way I used the right language at the right time. That changed the dynamic in the room.

It did not mean I suddenly had all the answers, but it meant I could follow the conversation and make informed choices. It meant I could protect myself better and challenge misinformation when it came. It meant I could keep up. For a woman who had once sat in the car after appointments feeling lost, that was no small transformation.

If there is one thing I tell other patients now, it is this: you do not need a medical degree to learn how to advocate for yourself. You just need curiosity, persistence, and the courage to ask questions. The more you learn, the more confident you become. And the more confident you become, the harder it is for anyone to dismiss you.

Struggle

Medical jargon made me feel small, excluded, and shut out of conversations about my own body. I often left appointments confused, embarrassed, and afraid to ask questions because I did not want to sound uninformed. That confusion made me feel powerless.

Insight

I realized that clarity is not optional. If I did not understand what was being said, I could not truly participate in my care. Learning the language of medicine did not make me a doctor, but it helped me become an informed partner in the room instead of a passive bystander.

Lesson

Understanding is your right. Clarity is part of good care, not a bonus.

Guidance

A few things that helped me learn the language of my care:

- When you hear unfamiliar terms, write them down and look them up later.
- Ask directly: "Can you explain that in plain English?"
- Repeat back what you think you heard and ask, "Is that correct?"
- Keep a running glossary in your journal of medical terms, lab names, and diagnoses.
- Do not leave the room confused just because you are afraid of asking too many questions.
- Remember that understanding your care is not being difficult; it is being responsible.

The more clearly you understand what is happening, the more confidently you can respond to it.

CHAPTER 9

When They Don't Believe You

One of the hardest parts of living with chronic illness is not always the pain itself. Sometimes it is the constant battle to be believed. Pain is exhausting. Symptoms are frightening. Uncertainty alone can wear you down. But there is another layer of suffering people do not always talk about: the emotional and psychological toll of explaining what is happening in your body, only to be met with doubt, dismissal, or that subtle look that says, I'm not sure I believe you.

That kind of response leaves its own kind of bruise.

When your body does not fit neatly into a diagnosis, when your symptoms do not show up clearly on a test, or when your condition is complicated enough that it resists easy explanations, some doctors begin looking at you as if the problem must not be in your body at all. They act as if the pain must be exaggerated, the symptoms must be emotional, or as if the issue is not the illness but your interpretation of it.

I have lost count of how many times I have sat in an exam room describing what I was feeling only to be met with a raised eyebrow, a half-smile, a quick shrug, or the phrase so many patients have come to dread: "It's probably just stress."

Now let me be clear: stress is real. Stress affects the body and can absolutely make health problems worse. But there is a difference between acknowledging the role of stress and using stress as a lazy explanation for pain that deserves a proper evaluation. Too often, "stress" becomes the escape hatch. It is the quick answer when a provider does not know and the convenient label when they do not feel like digging deeper. It is the neat little box they place you in when your body is asking questions they are not prepared to answer.

When that happens repeatedly, it can start to get in your head. You begin to wonder if maybe you did explain it wrong. Maybe you sounded too emotional. Maybe you should have used different words. Maybe you are overreacting, tired, or imagining the severity of what you feel. That is part of what makes medical dismissal so dangerous. It does not just deny your experience in the moment; it can slowly teach you to distrust yourself.

One particular moment still stings when I think about it. I had been seeing a pain management doctor for years. He knew my history and my struggles. He knew the endless list of tests, medications, procedures, and appointments I had already endured. He was not new to my case. He had watched me walk through enough to know that I was not someone casually inventing symptoms or dramatizing my pain.

So when I came to him one day with chest pain—pain we already knew was not heart-related—I thought he would take me seriously. It was not because I expected instant answers, but because I expected thoughtful attention. I expected curiosity. I expected him to approach the pain as something worth respecting, even if it did not fit neatly into a familiar explanation.

Instead, after doing a few quick checks and finding nothing obvious, he leaned back and said, "Sometimes stress manifests itself as pain. Maybe this is just stress or in your mind."

I laughed. I did not laugh because it was funny. I laughed because sometimes absurdity is so sharp that laughter is the only thing standing between you and tears.

"Stress?" I asked him. "You think I don't know the difference between stress and pain that knocks me to my knees?"

That question came from a place much deeper than irritation. It came from years of living in my body. It came from years of knowing what stress felt like and years of knowing what true physical pain felt like. I knew the difference between emotional strain and pain so intense it dropped me to my knees. But he did not answer. He had already moved on.

That may have been one of the hardest parts. It was not just what he said, but how quickly he said it and how little room there was afterward for anything else. There was no real pause and no deeper conversation. There was no acknowledgment of what it meant for a doctor I had trusted to so casually reduce my pain to something vague and dismissible. He had already decided. He was already mentally ending the visit.

Just like that, I was no longer a patient in need of care. I was a problem he had finished with.

I walked out of that appointment with tears burning in my eyes. I was hurting physically, but I was also hurting emotionally in a way that is hard to explain unless you have lived it. This was not a stranger brushing me off. This was someone I had trusted, someone who had been part of my care, and someone with enough context to know better.

There is a special kind of grief in realizing that a person you trusted medically does not actually trust you in return.

My son Chad was waiting downstairs in the car for me. The moment I got in, with tears already falling, he knew the appointment had not gone well. I did not have the energy to explain it. My mind was overwhelmed, my heart was heavy, and all I could do was cry. I went home carrying that ache with me.

At first, I replayed the conversation in my head the way patients so often do after a bad appointment. I thought about what I said, what I should have said, and what I wish I had said. I thought about the look on his face, the tone in his voice, and the way the conversation shut down instead of opening up. I thought about how much emotional energy it takes to keep showing up honestly in those rooms, only to be treated like your honesty is the problem.

But after the shock wore off, clarity came. I knew what I had to do. I reached out, but ended up speaking with one of the residents instead. Sometimes I think the doctor knew exactly why I called, and that may be why he never responded. But I needed him to know what that moment had cost me. I needed him to understand that what he said was not harmless. Telling a chronically ill patient that their pain is "just stress" without proper care or compassion does real damage.

Ending that relationship was painful, but it was necessary. Staying with a doctor who did not believe me was far more dangerous than the inconvenience of starting over with someone new.

That is one of the brutal truths of chronic illness: sometimes you have to grieve people before you are fully ready to let them go. Sometimes that includes doctors too. Sometimes the people you hoped would walk with you to the next stage of healing turn out not to be safe enough to keep on your team. When that happens, leaving is not disloyal; it is wise.

Being dismissed over and over again wears you down in ways people do not always see. It exhausts your spirit and chips away at your confidence, your clarity, and even your sense of reality. It can make you wonder whether maybe you ask for too much, feel too much, or expect too much.

But I have learned this: the voice inside me, the one that knows when something is wrong, is not to be ignored. I may not have the letters "M.D." after my name, but I live in this body every single day. I know its patterns. I know its warnings. I know when something is familiar and when something is different. I know the difference between discomfort and danger, between stress and pain that takes my breath away.

That knowledge matters. It may not replace a diagnosis or testing. It may not answer every question, but it matters. I have learned to treat it with respect, even when others do not.

For every doctor who does not believe you, there is one who will. It may take time to find them. It may take persistence, trial and error, disappointment, and courage. It may take walking away from people you once trusted. It may take more explaining and more paperwork than you ever wanted. But you still deserve that doctor.

You deserve a provider who takes you seriously. You deserve someone who honors your experience. You deserve care that does not begin from suspicion. You deserve a medical relationship where your body is not treated like a debate.

To anyone who has ever sat in an exam room feeling small, belittled, or quietly shattered by the implication that it is "all in your head," I want you to hear this clearly: You are not imagining it. Your pain deserves to be taken seriously. Your experience matters. And your voice does too. Being disbelieved hurts, but it is not the truth of your body.

Struggle

One of the deepest struggles in chronic illness is not only the pain itself, but the damage that comes from being doubted. Having to explain what is happening in your body over and over, only to be met with dismissal, can wear down your confidence and distort your sense of reality. When doctors reduce real pain to "just stress" without truly listening, it does not only delay care. It can make you question yourself. It can make you wonder whether you explained it wrong, felt too much, or expected too much. That kind of disbelief wounds more than trust. It can leave you feeling emotionally stranded inside your own body.

Insight

I learned that being disbelieved hurts, but it is not the truth of my body. A doctor's doubt does not cancel out what I know I am feeling. I may not have every medical answer, but I live in this body every day. I know its patterns, its warnings, and the difference between ordinary stress and pain that signals something is wrong. I also learned that trust in healthcare must go both ways. If a provider does not respect my lived experience, they are not a safe place for my care.

Guidance

A few things this experience taught me:

- Pay attention to how a provider responds when you describe pain. Dismissal, minimization, or condescension are warning signs.
- If someone says it is "just stress," ask what has been ruled out and what evaluation supports that conclusion.
- Write down statements that feel dismissive, especially if they affect treatment decisions.
- Do not ignore your own knowledge of your body just because someone with authority seems certain.
- If a doctor repeatedly makes you feel small, unbelieved, or unsafe, it is okay to leave and find someone else.
- Being emotional does not make your symptoms less real. Pain is still pain, even when it comes with frustration, fear, or tears.
- Keep looking for the provider who listens with both skill and respect.

And if you want a closing line in the same tone as your other chapters, use this:

Being disbelieved may wound your spirit, but it does not define the truth of what your body is carrying.

CHAPTER 10

Building Your Support Circle

When chronic illness enters your life, it does not just affect you. It reshapes everything around you. It changes your routines, your energy, your plans, your priorities, your relationships, and sometimes even the way your home functions from day to day. Tasks most people take for granted, such as cooking, cleaning, driving, lifting a child, walking into an appointment, or even getting dressed, can suddenly feel overwhelming or impossible. Things you once did without thinking can begin to require planning, help, and more energy than you have to give.

That is when your circle of support becomes not just helpful, but essential.

I learned this early. After my first major health crisis, I had to come face to face with a truth I did not want to admit: I could not do this alone. As much as I wanted to be independent and as much as I wanted to keep functioning the way I always had, my body had changed the rules. There were days when I needed help with the simplest parts of life.

And that was hard for me.

I had always taken pride in handling things. I was the one who showed up. I was the one who figured it out. I was the one who made a way. So needing help did not feel natural to me. It felt painful. It felt humbling. It felt, at times, like failure. But illness has a way of stripping away the illusion that independence is the highest form of strength. It taught me that survival often depends on letting other people step close enough to carry what you cannot carry alone.

And thank God, I had people who did. My close friends became part of the village that carried me when I could not carry myself.

Cliff and Nikki, who are Kaitlyn's godparents, stepped in in one of the most important ways possible. They became caregivers for my baby girl when I could not be there the way I wanted to be. When I was hospitalized and separated from her, they made sure she was not only cared for, but loved. There is no way to fully explain what that meant to me as a mother. Knowing that my baby was safe in the hands of people who truly loved her gave me peace in moments that otherwise would have broken me. Their help was not small; it was sacred.

And then there was Carol, Kaitlyn's godmother. When Kaitlyn was born, I was so sick that I could not go home even though my baby had to leave the hospital, and that was one of the most heartbreaking moments of my life. But Carol and her family stepped in without hesitation, taking my baby girl home and caring for her with tenderness, love, and selflessness until I was well enough to come home too. What Carol did revealed a rare kind of friendship and love, the kind that shows up quietly, sacrificially, and without being asked twice, and even after that season she continued showing up for Kaitlyn whenever possible. I will always be grateful for the way she helped carry us through one of the most painful moments of my early motherhood.

Joan was also part of that village. She loved Kaitlyn in such a beautiful and generous way. She took care of her and even took her along on her travels as she performed across the United States. That kind of love is extraordinary. It was not just babysitting; it was giving my daughter joy, care, consistency, and experiences in a season when so much of life felt uncertain. Joan helped make sure Kaitlyn's world did not shrink just because mine had.

Then there was Owen. Owen made sure Chad and Kaitlyn had food in the house at all times, which was no small thing when I was in and out of the hospital and so much of life felt unstable. He also brought them to see me. He helped keep that connection alive between us when hospital walls threatened to make everything feel distant. Those acts may sound simple on paper, but they were not simple at all. They were acts of steady, practical love. It was the kind of love that says, "You do not have to figure out every detail by yourself." And that kind of love matters deeply in a crisis.

There was my friend Kesta who showed up for me in ways I will always remember. He took me to appointment after appointment, rushed me to the emergency room when needed, and made sure I had company and was eating well during my hospital stays. He showed up with consistency, loyalty, and care. In the world of chronic illness, dependability is one of the greatest gifts anyone can give you, and he gave that gift generously. He was not just helping me get from place to place. He was helping me carry the weight of a life that had become medically complicated, emotionally exhausting, and deeply uncertain.

Stephanie was my aide at the time, but over the years she became one of my closest friends. She went above and beyond in ways I will never forget. What she did for Kaitlyn was never really part of her job description, but love rarely stops to check titles before it shows up. She cared for Kaitlyn with a tenderness, patience, and dependability that blessed me deeply. In time, she became much more than an aide. She became a dear friend and one of the people who helped carry me through some of the hardest moments of this journey.

My church family became another powerful layer of support around us. They prayed for me, checked on me, helped hold my family together, and made sure Kaitlyn was surrounded with love, normalcy, and joy. They picked her up for church, took her to dinner, and took her on playdates. My church sisters even braided her hair so Chad would not have to carry one more thing while I was in the hospital. Their love was practical, tender, and steady. It reminded me over and over again that we were not walking through that season alone.

Our local library also became a safe place for Kaitlyn during a season when her young life was filled with fear, confusion, and uncertainty. Every week, she would spend time there doing crafts, playing games, and finding a little escape from the complicated reality she was growing up in. When I was too sick to bring her, Stephanie would take her or the library would call and offer to pick her up and drop her off. That kindness was a blessing we never expected. They cared for my baby girl with such tenderness that even now, it sometimes brings me to tears thinking about how they looked out for her.

My son Chad was almost twenty when my health began to spiral. He became the son and big brother I had prayed for. Instead of living only for himself in that season of life, he stepped up in ways that still humble me when I think about them. He took care of his baby sister as if she were his own child. He became her main caregiver while I was in the hospital, carrying responsibilities that many young men his age could not have handled with that kind of grace.

There is something both beautiful and heartbreaking about that truth. It was beautiful because of the love in it, but heartbreaking because as a mother, I never wanted my son to have to grow up so fast or carry that kind of weight so young. But Chad did. He showed up. He protected her. He nurtured her. He helped hold our family together. And he did it with a steadiness that still takes my breath away. He was not just helping out; he was carrying us. That kind of love changes a family forever.

My daughter Kaitlyn, though only a baby when all of this began, also grew up inside the reality of having a mom who was sick. She did not get the kind of childhood untouched by hospitals, emergencies, and sudden change. There were days when I would leave home for what was supposed to be a simple doctor's appointment and not return for weeks because I was rushed to the hospital and admitted. She saw hospital rooms, machines, and the painful reality that life could change quickly.

But she also saw love. She saw people show up. She saw what community looks like when it wraps itself around a family in crisis. Through all of it, she grew into compassion and resilience far beyond her years. As she got older, she quietly became part of my care team too. She did it not in grand dramatic ways, but in the small, tender ways that children often do. She offered comfort, she made me laugh, and she brought light into dark seasons. She reminded me with her love why I kept fighting.

The love of my children, my friends, my church family, and the people God placed around me carried me through seasons that I never could have survived by strength alone. And that taught me something important: support is not extra. It is not a luxury. It is part of care.

But in building my support circle, I also had to come to terms with something else: I was grieving the fact that I could not take care of myself the way I once had. I had always been an independent person, and now my life had been reduced to needing someone to bathe me, wash my hair, feed me, help me out of bed, and help care for my child. Even when the help was loving and gentle, there was still pain in needing it.

It has been a struggle. Over the years, though, with the help of my amazing doctors and the support of the people around me, I have been able to reclaim some of that independence. In the last couple of years, I have started driving again locally, here and there. That may sound small to some people, but for me it is major. Being able to cook with help instead of not at all, take a walk around the block without feeling like my body is on fire, or participate in my church—those are things most people take for granted. When illness is all you have known for so long, those things become significant. They become victories.

And yes, I am in severe pain every single day. But because I am so grateful for getting another chance to be here, I tend to go hard and go all in. Sometimes that means my health takes a turn for the worse. Sometimes it means I pay for it afterward. But sometimes it is worth it just to see the impact on the lives of others, to be present, and to feel useful. It is worth it to feel alive in a way illness cannot completely steal.

That, too, is part of the tension of this life. It is being grateful to be here while still grieving what has been lost. It is pushing forward while knowing there may be a cost. It is wanting to live fully while living in a body with limits.

I am blessed to have people I can trust. Not everyone has that, and I know that. Support comes in different forms, and for my family it has often looked like love wrapped in comfort and peace. It feels amazing to have that kind of support. And at the same time, it has been painful because I needed it. That is the complicated truth. Support can feel like grace and grief at the same time.

Not everyone begins with a village already formed around them. If that is your truth, I want to say gently that it does not mean you cannot build one. Support circles are not always automatic. Sometimes they have to be created.

Sometimes they begin with one person or one honest conversation. Sometimes they begin with the humbling decision to stop pretending you are fine when you are not.

For me, building support required letting go of pride. And that was not easy. I had to learn, slowly and painfully, that needing help did not make me weak. It made me human. It made me honest. It made me someone living inside real limitations instead of denying them. Once I finally admitted that I could not do it all, I made room for people to step in.

And many of them did.

I also learned that building a support circle means being specific. People often want to help, but they do not know how. They may care deeply and still feel unsure of what would actually be useful. That is why vague requests can leave both sides frustrated. Saying "I need help" matters, but saying "Can you bring a meal on Thursday?" or "Can you take me to this appointment?" gives people something concrete to say yes to.

Specific asks create practical support, and practical support saves energy. That mattered for me because chronic illness already takes so much. It takes your energy, your time, your flexibility, your privacy, and often your sense of normalcy. The people around you should not drain you further. They should steady you. They should help refill what illness keeps pouring out.

That does not mean everyone in your circle has to do everything. It just means your support system should be made up of trustworthy people. You need people who show up, people who do not make your hardest moments about themselves, and people who do not guilt you for needing help. You need people who bring peace instead of chaos.

Your circle does not have to be large. It does not have to look impressive from the outside. Sometimes one or two dependable people are more life-giving than a crowd full of noise. What matters is consistency. What matters is trust. What matters is knowing who you can call when the floor drops out from under you.

I would not have survived the past decade without my circle. That is not dramatic; it is true. They reminded me over and over again that while illness may limit the body, it does not limit love. Love, expressed through meals, rides, prayers, and practical help, became one of the ways God kept me going.

Sometimes healing comes through medicine. Sometimes it comes through surgery. Sometimes it comes through knowledge and advocacy. And sometimes it comes through the simple, sacred act of someone showing up and saying, "You do not have to carry this alone."

Struggle

Accepting help was painful for me. I had always been fiercely independent and proud of being able to manage on my own. So when illness forced me into situations where I needed help bathing, cooking, or caring for my children, it felt like a loss I did not know how to name. It touched my pride and challenged my identity. Even when support felt beautiful, I was still grieving the fact that I needed it.

Insight

Community is not weakness; it is resilience. My illness taught me that allowing others in was not surrender. It was survival. The people who showed up for me were not proof that I had failed; they were proof that I was loved. I also learned that support can feel like both comfort and grief at the same time. You can be deeply grateful for help and still mourn the independence you lost.

Lesson

Strength is not doing everything alone. Strength is knowing when to lean on others. And sometimes healing also means celebrating the small ways you reclaim pieces of your independence along the way.

Guidance

A few things that helped me build and lean on my support circle:

- Identify three to five people you can call in a crisis and let them know they are on your emergency list.
- Be specific when asking for help with meals, rides, note-taking, or childcare.
- Accept help without guilt. Often, the people who love you are grateful to be given a meaningful way to show it.
- Build support beyond family through church, trusted friends, neighbors, aides, or support groups.
- Keep a written list of who can help with what so you are not trying to figure it out in the middle of an emergency.
- Celebrate small gains in independence like driving locally, taking a walk, or cooking with help.
- Pay attention to who leaves you feeling lighter and who leaves you more drained. Choose your circle accordingly.

You do not need a huge village. You need a trustworthy one.

CHAPTER 11

When Your Body Becomes a Battlefield

There is something deeply unsettling about living in a body that no longer feels safe. A body is supposed to be your shelter. It is supposed to carry you through life, help you move, help you rest, and help you mother. Even when it is imperfect, you trust it in quiet ways without realizing you are trusting it at all. You trust your legs to hold you, your lungs to breathe, and your heart to beat. You trust that when you wake up in the morning, your body will at least be recognizable to you.

But chronic illness changes that relationship. It can turn your body from a home into a battlefield.

That is what happened to me. There came a point in this journey when I realized I was no longer just dealing with isolated symptoms or occasional emergencies. I was living inside an ongoing war. My body was not just hurting me from time to time; it was challenging me daily. Some days it felt like every system had joined the fight: my blood, my nerves, my joints, my skin, my energy, my stomach, my mind, my sleep, and my strength. Everything felt touched by the battle.

When your body becomes a battlefield, you grieve in ways people cannot always see. You grieve the body you used to have and the ease you once moved through life with. You grieve the woman you thought you would be and the simple trust you once had in your own flesh. That grief is real. It is not vanity or weakness. It is the pain of losing familiarity with yourself.

There is nothing like the pain of not being able to trust your body on any level. For me, that betrayal began when I was pregnant with Kaitlyn. I spent so much of that pregnancy in and out of the hospital that it felt like I was living in two worlds. One was trying to protect my baby and one was trying to survive what my body was doing. At one point, I even had my own baby monitoring machine. Between blood transfusions, infusion treatments, and the constant fight to keep both me and my baby alive, my body felt like it was failing me from every direction.

And yet, at the same time, it was also trying to be a protective space for my daughter. That tension has stayed with me. When I think back on that season, my body stopped feeling like something that belonged to me in the way it once had. It became a site of crisis but also a place of protection. It was fighting, failing, and carrying life all at once. There is something so complicated about that as a mother: to feel betrayed by your body and still need that same body to keep your child alive.

Once trust is broken inside your own skin, it is hard to fully recover that innocence. There have been mornings when I woke up so swollen and puffy that I barely recognized my own face. There have been days when my hands were so swollen and painful I could barely use them. There were days when I was so unstable on my feet that even walking felt uncertain, and days when I could not bathe myself. There were days when my body felt so heavy and exhausted that simply standing felt like too much.

One of the deepest struggles has been the change in my weight. I had always been a thin person, and that was the body I recognized as mine. Having to deal with my body nearly doubling in weight was not just physically difficult; it was emotionally devastating. It was not simply about numbers on a scale. It was about identity. It was about looking in the mirror and feeling like the person staring back at me was someone I did not know. Once the diagnoses kept coming, so did the medications, and with them came the weight. I understand there are medical reasons for it, but acceptance and pain are not always the same thing. Even now, the shame can still find me.

On any given day, the shame can still find me. I know I should not feel that way. I know my body has been through more than most people will ever understand and that it has fought hard to keep me here. But trauma leaves fingerprints. The body remembers. Sometimes no matter how much healing work you do or how much truth you know in your head, the emotional toll still lingers in the mirror.

Over the years, the mirror became my enemy. No matter how many people told me I looked great, I could not always receive it the way they meant it. There was a time when hearing "You look great" would trigger something in me that I could not move past. What the public saw and what I saw were two very different things. The public saw presentation. They saw clothes, hair, a smile, and effort. But at home, looking in the mirror was something I often avoided because I was seeing grief, medication, and trauma. I was seeing all the ways my life and body had changed without my permission.

Chronic illness is not just pain. It is disruption, interruption, and betrayal. Sometimes it feels like your own body is the thing you have to survive.

There were seasons when I felt angry at my body. I was angry that it could not do what I needed it to do and that it kept failing me in moments when I needed strength. I was angry that it required so much management just to function at a basic level. I was angry that I had to think so hard about what other people do without a second thought, such as eating, bathing, sleeping, walking, or just living.

When your body becomes a battlefield, even ordinary acts can feel loaded. Then there are the medications. People often hear the names and do not realize what they represent. These are just some of the many medications that have become part of my daily life:

ELIQUIS: A reminder that my blood has been dangerous enough that I need daily protection against clotting.

CYMBALTA: Part of trying to manage pain, nerve issues, and the emotional toll that comes with carrying physical suffering and mental strain.

DAPSONE: One more medication in the long line of treatments meant to quiet what my body keeps stirring up.

PLAQUENIL: A name that became part of daily life and the fight against inflammation and autoimmune complications.

PREDNISONE: A medication that can help but also comes with its own price. It brings swelling and the visible changes that make you look in the mirror and feel like your illness is wearing your face.

METHOTREXATE: A serious medication for a serious fight. It reminds you daily that this is not a minor struggle or something temporary.

FARXIGA: Added to help protect my kidneys and manage yet another layer of this complicated health journey.

Each of these medications tells part of the story. Each bottle represents a battle being fought inside me. Each dose is an act of maintenance, survival, hope, and frustration all at once. Medication is never just medication when you are chronically ill. It is also side effects, timing, stomach issues, brain fog, nausea, and inflammation. It is taking sixteen medications a day and still feeling some side effects as if it were your first dose.

There are days when it feels like I am taking medicine just to survive the effects of the medicine that is helping me survive. And yet, I keep taking it because that is what life on a battlefield looks like. You do what you have to do. You adapt. You learn the language of your own body. You become both student and soldier in your own survival.

But I want to say this clearly: there is an emotional cost to all of that. There is a cost to feeling like your body is always demanding something from you and a cost to never fully relaxing inside your own skin. There is a cost to not knowing which body will greet you when you wake up. Some days that cost looks like sadness or exhaustion so deep you cannot even explain it.

Then there were the lonely days and nights in the hospital. People see the hospital as the place where help is, and it is, but it can also be one of the loneliest places in the world. There were nights when the halls grew quiet, the machines kept beeping, and I was left there alone with the ache of being away from my children. There is a particular kind of pain that comes from lying in a hospital bed knowing your children are somewhere else sleeping without you.

At one point I refused to take pictures. It was easier that way. If I did not have to look at myself later, then I did not have to sit with the disconnect between who I felt I was and who the camera captured. But one day Kaitlyn looked at me and said, “Mom, please take pictures with me. I just want to make memories with you, and if anything happens to you, I won’t have many pictures of you.”

That broke me, and it healed something too. I realized that my children were not looking at me through the same harsh eyes I was using on myself. They were not measuring my worth by weight or swelling. They just wanted their mother. From that day forward, I never refused a photo with my children. Love began to speak louder than avoidance.

On one of my really bad days, Dr. Schlair told me, "Your only job is to survive today. That's your only job going forward." That landed in me deeply. When you are chronically ill, the world still expects you to perform as if nothing is wrong. But on that day, my doctor gave me permission to strip life all the way down to its most basic truth. Survival was enough.

I made the decision to show up for myself so that I could keep showing up for the people I love. Some days that meant taking my medicine and resting. Other days it meant admitting I could not do more than make it through the day. Showing up for myself was not selfish; it was necessary. My children needed me alive.

I stopped measuring strength only by how much I could push through. Sometimes strength looked like surviving the day, and that counted. Chronic illness can force you into a strange relationship with yourself. You may love your body because it is yours and still feel disappointed in it. You may care for it faithfully and still feel betrayed by it. I had to learn not to shame myself for grieving.

Grief did not make me ungrateful; it made me honest. And honesty matters when your body becomes a battlefield, because pretending everything is fine only deepens the loneliness of the fight. I also had to learn something tender: my body was not my enemy even when it felt like it.

My body was not trying to destroy me; it was struggling. It was carrying trauma, inflammation, pain, and exhaustion. It was not cooperating the way I wanted, but it was still carrying me the best it could under impossible circumstances. Once I stopped seeing my body only as a traitor, I could begin caring for it with more mercy, patience, and tenderness. I stopped demanding perfection from a body fighting multiple battles at once.

When your body becomes a battlefield, survival becomes deeply personal. It is about identity, grief, and dignity. It is about learning how to look at yourself with compassion even when you do not recognize the woman in the mirror. It is about refusing to let pain be the only narrator of your story.

My body has become a battlefield, but it is still my body. I am still here. I am still learning it, caring for it, and thanking God for it.

Struggle

One of the hardest parts of chronic illness is the emotional strain of living in a body that feels unpredictable and unfamiliar. Swelling, side effects, exhaustion, and significant weight gain can make you feel disconnected from yourself. There is grief and anger in waking up and not knowing what version of your body you will get. The lonely hospital nights away from my children deepened that pain. The battle is not only physical; it is emotional, mental, and spiritual too.

Insight

I learned that grief for my body did not make me weak or ungrateful. It made me honest. I also learned that survival is enough on the hardest days. When Dr. Schlair told me my only job was to survive today, she gave me permission to stop measuring myself by normal standards and start honoring what my life really required. Showing up for myself was one of the ways I could keep showing up for the people I love.

Lesson

When your body becomes a battlefield, treat it with honesty and mercy. You may need to fight for it, advocate for it, and grieve it, but do not abandon it. On the hardest days, survival is a worthy goal all by itself.

Guidance

A few things that helped me survive life in a body that felt unsafe:

- Name your grief honestly. Mourning what your body used to do is real and valid.
- Track medication side effects and speak up when the burden becomes too great.
- Do not force yourself to pretend you are fine when you are struggling.
- Practice speaking to your body with more compassion rather than more blame.
- Let support in when daily life becomes physically overwhelming.
- On the hardest days, narrow your focus to surviving today. Face tomorrow when it comes.
- Let love interrupt shame. Your children often see truth more clearly than your pain does.
- Remember that body changes, pain, and weight gain do not erase your dignity.

Your body may be fighting hard. That does not mean you stop being worthy of tenderness.

CHAPTER 12

The Power of Research

When you are first thrown into the world of illness, it is tempting to put all your trust in the professionals. After all, they are the ones with the degrees, the white coats, the training, and the access to language that often feels just out of reach. It would be easier, in some ways, to hand the whole thing over and believe that someone else will connect the dots, weigh the risks, and carry the burden of figuring it out.

But I learned early on that while doctors may have medical knowledge, I had lived experience. And those two things needed to work together.

At first, I was intimidated by research. I did not want to become "that patient." I did not want to be the one who shows up with printouts from the internet, the one doctors roll their eyes at before she has even sat down, or the one who sounds like she has diagnosed herself from a search engine at two in the morning. But after being dismissed, misdiagnosed, brushed off, and overlooked more times than I can count, I realized that research was not optional for me. It was part of survival.

So I began to read. I read articles, medical journals, condition-specific websites, patient forums, medication information sheets, and research summaries. I studied hospital pages and foundation websites. I studied not only diagnoses but side effects, drug interactions, lab values, and questions I should be asking.

I learned how to tell the difference between credible information and noise. That mattered. Because not all research is equal. Some information calms you, some empowers you, and some sends you spiraling. I had to learn not just how to research, but how to research wisely.

I started paying attention to the source. Was it from a reliable hospital or medical institution? Was it a peer-reviewed study? Was it a condition-specific organization or a patient group sharing lived experience that aligned with what I was seeing in my own body? I did not need to become a physician. I needed to become informed enough to ask sharper questions.

That shift changed everything. I remember nights sitting at the kitchen table long after everyone else had gone to bed. My notebook was full of scribbles and my laptop was open with tabs stacked across the screen. I was chasing language, patterns, and possibilities. I was not researching because I enjoyed it. I was researching because I was trying to understand a body that kept doing things no one seemed able to explain fast enough.

I was trying to survive.

There is a certain desperation in late-night research when you are sick. You are tired and scared. You are trying to make sense of symptoms, test results, and treatment options while still carrying the emotional weight of everything else. Because you are desperate for answers, the line between empowerment and overwhelm can get thin very quickly. I had to learn that too.

Research can become a rabbit hole if you are not careful. One article leads to another. One symptom leads to ten possibilities. One medication warning leads to twenty more fears. Before you know it, your body is still in pain and your mind is spiraling too.

There were times to dig deeper and there were times to close the laptop and breathe. There were times to bring what I found into the room and times to let it sit until I had more context. But what I never did again was let anyone make me feel ashamed for wanting to understand my own body.

Research paid off more than once. There were times when I walked into appointments armed with information that shifted the direction of my care. Once, I raised a concern about a medication adjustment based on research I had done around INR levels and clotting risk. My doctor paused, considered it seriously, and said, "That's a good point. Let's take a closer look."

That moment stayed with me. It reminded me that an informed patient is not a burden. An informed patient can be a partner. In complex medical journeys, partnership matters.

There were also times when research helped me recognize patterns before they were obvious to everyone else. When I saw medication side effects lining up with what I was experiencing, I could ask better questions. When I understood more about my diagnoses, I could describe my concerns more clearly. When I knew how a condition commonly progressed or what red flags to watch for, I could act more quickly instead of second-guessing myself.

Research did not replace the doctor, but it made me less dependent on blind trust. Blind trust can be dangerous in a system that is rushed, fragmented, and sometimes dismissive. Research gave me another layer of protection. It helped me recognize when something sounded off, when a treatment plan needed more questions, and when I needed to advocate with more confidence because I was speaking from both experience and information.

And that combination is powerful.

I also researched doctors. That became part of my process too. I wanted to know what people said about them, what hospital systems they worked with, and what their specialties were. I wanted to know what conditions they commonly treated and whether there were signs that they might actually understand the complexity I was living with. Online reviews do not tell the whole story, but they can sometimes give you clues about communication style and responsiveness. When you have already lived through enough dismissive care, those clues matter.

One of the most important things research gave me was language. It gave me words for what to ask, what to question, and what might need follow-up. It also gave me steadiness. Instead of walking into appointments feeling powerless, I walked in with notes, questions, and a better understanding of what was being discussed. I could ask smarter questions and follow the conversation more closely. I could hear the gaps more clearly. I could say, "I read this, does it apply to me?" instead of sitting there silently hoping the room would somehow produce clarity on its own.

I have learned that good research is not about fear; it is about preparation. It is about becoming informed enough to participate meaningfully in the decisions that affect your life. For me, that made a difference not only medically but emotionally. Every time I learned something useful, I felt a little less helpless. Every time I found language for what I was living with, I felt a little less alone and a little more grounded in the room.

That matters. Chronic illness can make you feel like your life is happening to you. Research was one of the ways I began taking some of that power back.

Struggle

At first, research overwhelmed me. There was too much information, too many contradictions, and too many rabbit holes that led to more anxiety than clarity. Some nights I closed the laptop feeling more afraid than when I opened it.

Insight

I learned that not all information is useful, and not all research is wise. The goal was never to become my own doctor. It was to become informed enough to ask better questions, recognize patterns, and participate more fully in my care.

Lesson

Knowledge is not a cure, but it is a tool. Research can help you walk into care with more clarity, confidence, and power.

Guidance

A few things that helped me research without drowning in it:

- Start with reliable sources like major hospitals, medical institutions, and condition-specific organizations.
- Keep a research journal with terms, questions, links, and notes.
- Bring what you learn into appointments by asking, "Does this apply to me?"
- Focus on research that helps you ask better questions rather than just worry more.
- Pay attention to source quality before trusting what you read.

- Know when to close the laptop and rest. Information overload is real.

Research is most helpful when it supports your care and not when it consumes your peace.

CHAPTER 13

Finding Your Voice

In the beginning, I was timid in exam rooms. I nodded politely, let doctors rush me, and often left with more questions than answers. I did not want to upset anyone. I did not want to be labeled difficult. I did not want to come across as emotional, combative, or ungrateful. I thought that if I was respectful enough, patient enough, and quiet enough, maybe I would be taken seriously.

But the longer I lived with chronic illness, the more I realized that silence could cost me my health and sometimes even my life. If I did not speak up, I risked being overlooked. If I did not ask the extra question, I risked leaving with half-answers and full confusion. If I did not correct what was wrong in the room, I risked letting someone else's assumptions take over my care.

Finding my voice was not easy. It came in small steps. It was the first time I interrupted a doctor to say, "Actually, I'm not done speaking." It was the first time I asked, "Can you explain that in plain English?" and the first time I walked out of an appointment and thought, *I was heard.*

Those moments mattered because they were not just about communication. They were about reclaiming some of the power illness had stripped away. They were about remembering that even though I was a patient, I was still a person. I was a person with instincts, questions, and rights. I was a person whose body was not public property just because it was being treated.

Over time, my voice grew stronger. I stopped apologizing for asking questions. I stopped shrinking when I was not taken seriously. I stopped letting fear keep me quiet. I learned to set goals before every appointment by asking: *What do I need to walk away with today?* I learned to prepare my questions ahead of time so I would not forget them once I was in the room. I learned to pause and repeat back instructions to make sure I understood. And I learned to say no.

I said no to treatments that did not feel right. I said no to doctors who dismissed me. I said no to vague explanations that did not match what I was experiencing and no to the idea that my voice did not matter.

But there is another side of this that people do not always talk about. When you push back as a patient, one of your first thoughts is often: Will I get better care or worse care because I spoke up? That fear is real. When you are vulnerable, in pain, and dependent on someone for answers, speaking up can feel risky. Many of us are conditioned to be "good patients," to not ask too many questions, not take up too much time, and not make anyone uncomfortable. Underneath all of that is a deeper fear: if I say too much, will I be labeled difficult?

I think many of us are conditioned to be "good patients." Usually that means do not complain too much, do not ask too many questions, and do not take up too much time. It means do not challenge the plan and do not make anyone uncomfortable. Smile, nod, and be grateful. Underneath all of that is a deeper fear: *if I say too much, will I be labeled difficult?*

That fear is not imaginary. For many of us, that fear is a response to medical gaslighting, dismissal, or past experiences where speaking up led to tension instead of care. The body remembers that too. By the time you enter the next exam room, part of you is already bracing for the emotional cost of telling the truth.

That is why finding your voice takes courage. It is not just about speaking. It is about speaking while afraid, uncertain, and vulnerable. It is about speaking while not feeling well and knowing the room may not always reward your honesty. And still, you choose to do it anyway.

What I had to keep reminding myself was this: I am the expert on my body. That does not mean I know everything medically or that I replace a doctor's training. It means I know what I feel, what has changed, what is worsening, and what is familiar versus what is not.

Speaking up is not about fighting your doctor. It is about giving them the information they need to do their job well. That shift in thinking helped me. When I stopped seeing advocacy as confrontation and started seeing it as necessary information-sharing, it became easier to speak. I began to understand that my silence did not protect me. It only protected everyone else from discomfort. My health was too important for that.

One of the best ways I learned to push back against fear was preparation. I learned to write down my three most important concerns before every appointment. That helps when nerves try to scatter your thoughts. Bring a friend, your adult child, or someone you trust to the appointment. That helps when you need another set of ears to ground you. Ask the doctor to slow down and explain things in plain language. That helps when the room starts moving faster than your body can keep up.

These things may sound simple, but they matter. Courage does not always show up in big dramatic speeches. Sometimes courage looks like a folded piece of paper with three questions on it. Sometimes courage looks like saying, "Can you slow down?" or telling the doctor, "That does not match my experience." It looks like not letting the visit end until the real concern has been addressed.

It takes a lot to push past the internal silence when you do not feel well or when you are hurting. It is hard when your emotions are already running high and your body feels fragile. But that is exactly why your voice matters. Vulnerability should not cancel your right to clarity. Pain should not erase your right to partnership. Fear should not be the thing making decisions about your care.

One of the most powerful shifts came when I realized my voice was not just for me. It was for my children too. Chad and Kaitlyn needed a mother who fought for herself and who modeled what it meant to advocate. They needed to see that being respectful does not mean being silent. They needed to learn that dignity and advocacy can live together.

In many ways, finding my voice reshaped my relationships with doctors. Some resisted it. They bristled when I pushed back or seemed irritated when I asked too many questions. They preferred a patient who nodded quietly and kept things moving. But the right doctors respected it. They welcomed it. They saw me not as a passive patient but as a partner.

That taught me something important: the right doctor will not punish you for having a voice. They may challenge you or educate you, but they will not make you feel small for wanting to understand what is happening inside your own body.

There is a kind of strength that comes when you stop waiting for permission to speak. You do not need to earn the right to be heard. You already have it. My voice may not always be loud, but it is steady and clear. And it is mine.

If you are reading this and struggling to find your own, start small. Write down one question and make sure you ask it. Correct a doctor when they interrupt you. Tell them when something does not feel right. Ask them to slow down and explain it in a way that makes sense. Bring someone with you if your fear makes it hard to hold the room alone.

Bit by bit, your voice will grow. One day, you will realize you no longer whisper. You speak with the authority of someone who knows her life depends on it.

Struggle

Finding my voice did not come overnight. It came after years of shrinking, apologizing, and accepting less than I deserved. Speaking up felt risky because I was afraid it would affect my care. I feared being labeled difficult or uncooperative. When you are already vulnerable, it is hard to challenge someone who seems to hold so much power over your recovery.

Insight

I realized that silence cost me more than discomfort. My body needed me to speak. My children needed me to survive. My fear, while valid, could not be the thing running the room. I also learned that advocacy is not about fighting the doctor; it is about giving them the truth they need in order to care for me properly.

Lesson

Advocacy is using your voice, even when it shakes, to insist on the truth of your experience. You do not have to be loud to be clear, and you do not have to feel fearless to speak.

Guidance

A few things that helped me find and use my voice:

- Write down your top three concerns before every appointment.
- Lead with the most important issue first instead of saving it for the end.

- Bring a trusted person with you when possible.
- Ask the doctor to slow down and explain things in plain language.
- Use simple phrases like: "That doesn't match my experience," "Can you explain why?" or "I'm not comfortable leaving without addressing this."
- Remember that fear after medical gaslighting is valid, but it does not mean you should stay silent.
- Practice speaking up in small ways. Voice grows with use.

Your voice matters. The more you use it, the stronger it becomes.

CHAPTER 14

Advocacy in Action

Advocacy is not just an idea. It is a practice. It lives in the smallest details and the biggest decisions. It shows up in the notebook you bring to every appointment, the courage to ask one more question, the decision to switch doctors, and the insistence on a second opinion. It shows up in the moments when you are tired, frustrated, or afraid, and still choose not to let your voice disappear.

For me, advocacy became part of my daily routine. I kept a medical journal where I wrote down everything: symptoms, pain levels, side effects, medication changes, the time of day things happened, what made them worse, and what made them better. What started as scribbles became one of my greatest tools. When doctors asked, "When did this start?" or "How has it changed?" I could open my notebook and give exact details. That record made it harder for anyone to dismiss me because I was not relying only on memory. I was walking in with evidence.

Advocacy also meant preparing before each appointment. I walked in with written questions, not trusting myself to remember everything once I was in the room. I set goals before every visit by asking what I needed from the appointment and what I wanted answered before I left.

That preparation mattered because when appointments felt rushed, my notes helped me stay focused instead of getting swallowed by the doctor's pace.

Sometimes advocacy meant saying something uncomfortable. It was the time I stopped a doctor mid-sentence and said, "Before we move forward, I need you to listen to me." It was the times I asked for plain English because I refused to leave more confused than when I came in. It was the moments I said, "That doesn't match what I'm experiencing." Advocacy meant refusing to be passive, even when passivity would have been easier.

It also meant protecting my own boundaries. There were times when I said no to treatments that did not feel right, even when there was pressure to just go along with the plan. I asked for alternatives, pushed for more testing, and refused to settle for quick explanations that did not actually address what was happening in my body.

And sometimes, advocacy meant filing a complaint when a doctor's behavior crossed the line. That was never about revenge; it was about accountability. It was about making sure no one else would be treated the way I had been.

Over time, advocacy stopped being something I did only in emergencies. It became a way of living, a lens through which I approached my care, my family, my community, and even my conversations with strangers. Once you learn how much is at stake when people are not heard, you begin to understand that advocacy reaches beyond your own body.

I cannot tell you how many emails and messages I have received from people who saw me on social media and reached out to ask questions about illness, doctors, or how to advocate for themselves. That still humbles me. People are hungry for help, language, and someone to say, "You are not crazy, and here is how you can speak up."

Sometimes the questions are simple and sometimes they are desperate. Answering those messages may seem small, but it is part of what advocacy looks like for me now. I take what I have learned and pour it back into others who are desperate for help. What I have survived has given me language and tools, and I feel called to use that in service of other people.

That is my lifestyle now. Advocacy is no longer just what I do in exam rooms; it is how I move through the world. And sometimes advocacy has shown up in moments I never expected.

I remember a time when I was admitted to the hospital and one of my nurses came into the room looking like something was wrong. We had built a relationship over time, so when I asked her what was going on, she told me she had been having stomach pain for a while but had not made time to get it checked. I was stunned. I looked at her and said, "You work in a hospital. What would it take for you to just get it checked out?"

She brushed it off and told me she did not want people from the hospital in her business. That stayed with me. The next day, I asked if she had time for a quick conversation on her break. I told her how important it was for her to put herself first. I told her that caring for everybody else meant very little if she ignored what her own body was trying to tell her. Then I asked her to do me a favor: get it checked out for me. I said, "Do it for me, and next time I see you, tell me what they said."

A few days later, she came back and told me she had made an appointment. I was so happy for her. She asked if she could hug me, and of course I gave her the biggest hug. Then I went home.

About a month later, I was back in the hospital again. I did not see her. That was when I was told that she had been diagnosed with terminal stomach cancer and had gone back to her home country to be with her family. The next time I came back, I was told she had passed away. They were doing a memorial service for her, and I was invited to attend because of the role I had played in encouraging her to finally get checked.

I cannot tell you how hard I cried. It hurt me to my core and opened something in me that I still carry. Here was a nurse, a woman who worked inside the system meant to promote health, and even she did not feel safe enough to get herself checked. She delayed. She put everyone else first.

How many more women has this happened to? How many ignore their pain because they do not have time? How many fear a system that is supposed to help heal them?

That moment taught me that advocacy is not always about you. Sometimes it looks like convincing someone else to put themselves first. Sometimes it looks like borrowing your voice until another woman can find her own. Even when the result is not what you wanted, it still matters that you spoke.

That nurse's story hurt me deeply, but it also sharpened my understanding of what advocacy means. Advocacy is not a guaranteed rescue and it does not always change the ending, but it can change the moment. It can interrupt delay and prompt action.

Advocacy also shows up in the ordinary rhythms of life. It looks like making sure I understand a medication before I take it, reading up on side effects, asking for plain-language explanations, demanding testing when my body is telling me something is wrong, and refusing to leave confused.

I have learned that advocacy is both proactive and reactive. It is proactive when you track symptoms and prepare questions. It is reactive when you push back or ask for a second opinion. Both matter, and both protect your health.

Advocacy is not just for the doctor's office. It is in the pharmacy when you ask about side effects. It is in the hospital when you double-check medications. It is in conversations with family when you explain your limits. Advocacy in action is messy, imperfect, and tiring, but it is also powerful.

It reminds you that while you may not control your illness, you do have power in how you respond to it: in the questions you ask, the boundaries you set, the care you refuse, and the records you keep. That power can make the difference between being overlooked and being cared for.

Struggle

Putting advocacy into action is intimidating. There is always the fear of being labeled difficult or dramatic, especially for women of color. I had to unlearn years of conditioning that taught me to stay quiet and be polite in medical spaces. Advocacy is also exhausting. It takes energy to track, prepare, and question while you are already in pain.

Insight

I learned that advocacy is not confrontation; it is partnership. It is standing firmly in truth, even if your voice shakes, and refusing to hand over your power just because someone else has a degree. I also learned that advocacy is bigger than my own life. What I have learned can become a lifeline for other people.

Lesson

Your advocacy can shift not only your care, but the care of the people around you. Sometimes the most powerful thing you can do is speak up for yourself, for your children, or for another woman who is still trying to find her voice.

Guidance

A few ways advocacy can become part of your daily life:

- Prepare questions ahead of time and bring them in writing.
- Role-play hard conversations with a trusted friend so your voice feels more ready.
- Use calm, assertive language such as: "I hear you, but here's what I am experiencing."
- Ask for plain-language explanations when medical jargon feels confusing.
- Learn about new medications before taking them, especially side effects.
- Push for testing when your body is telling you something is wrong.
- Answer others with compassion when they reach out for help.
- Remember that helping someone else put themselves first is also advocacy.

Sometimes advocacy is about saving your own life. Sometimes it is about reminding someone else that theirs matters too.

CHAPTER 15

Navigating the Healthcare System as a Black Woman

This has been one of the most frustrating parts of my entire journey. As a woman, it is hard enough to be seen and heard in the healthcare system. But as a Black woman, it is even harder. That is not bitterness talking; that is lived experience.

Too often, this system does not feel built to truly care for us. It feels more like a system that keeps us trapped in cycles of sickness, dismissal, and delay. Our concerns are brushed aside, our pain is minimized, and our symptoms are questioned. Somehow, there is still this dangerous undercurrent in medicine suggesting that Black women feel pain differently, tolerate more, or do not deserve the same urgency and tenderness.

The statistics back up what we feel in our bones. Research consistently shows that Black patients are less likely to receive adequate pain medication than white patients for the same conditions. In fact, a landmark study found that nearly half of first- and second-year medical students held at least one false biological belief about biological differences between Black and white people, including the idea that Black people have "thicker skin" or "less sensitive nerve endings."

I have felt that in exam rooms. I have had doctors ask me if I was sure about what I was feeling as if I did not live in my own body every day. When my answer was not what they wanted to hear, I would often get that little "hmm," that silence, or that look that says more than words ever could. That silence can be loud. So can a smirk or a raised eyebrow. It makes you feel like your pain has to audition to be believed.

I have left appointments crying, hurt, disappointed, and angry. That is the heaviest part of navigating healthcare as a Black woman. You are not only carrying the illness; you are carrying the burden of trying to be believable. You have to speak up, but not too strongly. You have to advocate, but not in a way that gets you labeled "difficult." It is exhausting.

I remember one appointment with a neurologist that still bothers me. I went to see him because my hands would swell and my right hand would take on a blue tint. During the appointment, while he was examining me, my right hand started swelling right there in front of his eyes. Then it started turning bluish. He saw it happen.

After a while, the color came back, he finished his testing, and I left. For once, I felt hopeful. I thought a doctor had finally seen what I had been trying to explain. I thought there would now be a clear record in my chart. But the next day, I checked my after-visit summary and there was nothing there.

Even though he had witnessed it himself, he chose not to put it in my chart. When I messaged him, he said he was not sure what he was looking at, so he did not document it. That does not make sense to me. If you witness something abnormal, why would you not document it?

Harmful care is not only cruelty; sometimes it is omission. Sometimes it is the decision not to write down what happened because it does not fit neatly into the provider's certainty. But when you do not document what you witness, you erase evidence.

Yet, in the middle of all of that, there were also moments when certain doctors restored my faith. Dr. Sheira Schlair was an absolute Godsend. She did not just treat me like a complicated case; she treated me like a whole person. She started an email thread with all of my doctors so everyone could stay on the same page. She made sure I was not left carrying the story alone. I know for a fact that not all of them were happy about it. I would walk into an appointment and hear, "Oh, I got an email from your doctor yesterday," usually with a smirk. But Dr. Schlair did not care. She was my biggest advocate.

She once called me from her own family vacation because she saw an urgent message I sent in MyChart. I bawled like a baby because I felt cared for. Not processed, but cared for.

Another doctor who stands out is my vascular surgeon. He saved my arm when it first turned blue. Even when his office no longer took my insurance, he still saw me because his main concern was keeping me alive. He once told me how much he worried about my case. I felt seen, not as a burden, but as a person whose life mattered.

So this chapter holds two truths at once: the system is broken, and there are still good doctors in it.

Healing care looks like listening, documenting what you see, and supporting the patient instead of silencing her. I believe that many doctors do want to help, but they are thrown into a system that pressures them to become servants of numbers. It becomes a revolving door. Humanity gets squeezed out unless a clinician fights to keep it.

That is why accountability matters. Black and Brown women continue to face a healthcare system where structural racism and socioeconomic realities lead to poorer outcomes. For example, Black women are three to four times more likely to die from pregnancy-related causes than white women, regardless of their income or education level.

Until the system changes, we keep speaking. We keep documenting. We keep asking questions. We do not stay with doctors who are not a good fit. That is not disloyal or rude; it is wisdom. If a doctor makes you feel small or treats your pain like a debate, you are allowed to walk away. You are allowed to build a care team that does not require you to shrink in order to receive help.

Navigating this system as a Black woman requires discernment and courage. It requires holy stubbornness. You are not asking for too much by wanting to be heard. You are asking for what should have been there all along.

Struggle

One of the greatest struggles was carrying the added burden of being a Black woman in a system that too often doubts or overlooks us. I was not only fighting illness; I was fighting assumptions and skepticism. That burden is exhausting and can leave you wounded long after the appointment is over.

Insight

I learned that the system may be broken, but I do not have to stay with providers who reflect that brokenness back onto me. The right doctor can make an enormous difference. Dr. Schlair and my vascular surgeon reminded me that healing care does exist.

Lesson

Do not be afraid to change doctors if they are not a good fit for you. Staying with someone who dismisses you is far more dangerous than starting over with someone who might actually hear you.

Guidance

A few things I learned about navigating healthcare as a Black woman:

- Pay attention to how a doctor makes you feel. Seen? Dismissed? Rushed? Your body often knows before your mind admits it.
- Do not ignore patterns of minimization or omission.
- Bring documentation and support people. Preparation helps protect you.
- If something happens in the room, ask for it to be documented clearly in your chart.
- Value doctors who invite partnership and treat you with dignity.
- Remember that wanting compassionate care is not asking for special treatment; it is asking for the standard you deserve.

The system may not always be built with us in mind, but that does not mean we stop insisting on being seen.

CHAPTER 16

The Mental Health Battle

Chronic illness does not just live in the body. It takes root in the mind and spirit too. It settles into your thoughts, your emotions, your sleep, and your plans for the future. It changes more than how you feel physically; it changes how you carry each day. It changes how much uncertainty your nervous system has to hold and how often you have to pretend to be okay when you are anything but.

That kind of weight adds up. The endless cycle of appointments, symptoms, and fear wears on you in ways that are hard to explain to people who have never lived inside it. There are days when the physical pain is sharp, but the emotional pain cuts even deeper. There are days when what hurts most is not what your body is doing, but what your life has become because of it.

I had to learn that caring for my mental health was just as important as treating my physical conditions. But I did not learn that easily. At first, I resisted. I thought I should be able to push through on my own. I thought being strong meant enduring quietly. I thought if I just prayed harder or held on longer, maybe I could outrun the emotional cost of what I was living through..

But I could not. And the truth is, chronic illness is isolating. It can leave you feeling trapped inside a body that will not cooperate. It can make you grieve the life you thought you would have and the version of yourself you used to be. It can make you terrified of the future because you no longer trust what tomorrow will ask of your body or your family.

There is a grief in all of that. It is a grief for your health, your independence, your energy, and your plans. When grief lives beside pain long enough, it can start to feel like depression.

Another layer of my mental health battle began long before some of the biggest medical crises fully unfolded. My stepmother died in September 2008, and her loss broke me in ways I still struggle to explain. Outside of my children, she was the person I loved most. But I never really had the time to grieve her. Almost immediately after her death, I was thrown into survival mode, and in many ways, I have been there ever since.

Missing her became its own kind of trauma. There were so many times I felt that if she were still here, somehow her love would have kept me whole. Even though I had siblings, her death left me feeling like I no longer had a family. I had lost my person. Because I was the stepchild, there were moments when her death made me feel like I no longer mattered. In the middle of all that turmoil, I realized I had to create a new sense of family for myself and for my children.

I remember one season when I was especially sick and we truly did not know what would happen. My son's grandmother, Marjorie, called me and said words I have never forgotten. She told me that if anything happened to me, they would take care of Chad and Kaitlyn, and I did not need to worry. She told me to focus on fighting and healing. She said their whole family had me, that they loved me, and that I was like a daughter to her.

That kind of love held me together. People showed up for me and my children again and again. There were so many times I spiraled because the fear of not being here for my children was unbearable. How do you prepare your children for that? How do you carry that fear and still pretend life is normal?

Emotionally, I was a wreck. And yet, every day God saw fit to give me another chance at life, I tried to live it in a meaningful way. Yes, I put on the happy face. But underneath that was a woman carrying grief, fear, trauma, and love all at the same time.

Therapy became a lifeline for me. That is not an exaggeration. My therapist gave me space to say the things I did not feel free to say anywhere else. In that room, I could tell the truth without trying to make it sound prettier than it really was. I could say that I was tired, angry, and scared. I could say that asking for help did not mean I was weak; it meant I was wise enough to know I could not carry it alone.

There were seasons when once-a-week therapy was not enough. On my hardest weeks, I reached out for extra sessions. Sometimes it was just a phone call or a quick text. Those small touches of support steadied me. There are seasons when what saves you is not one huge breakthrough, but the small, faithful supports that keep you from going under.

Faith anchored me too. Prayer gave me words when I had none. There were moments when I could not even form a polished prayer, but I could still cry out to God from the middle of my pain. Sometimes all I had was exhaustion and tears, and somehow even that became prayer. Scripture reminded me that I was not alone and that God did not need me polished to be near me. Worship helped too. It was a way to remember that my pain was not the only thing true about me.

Still, I will not pretend it was easy. There were nights I cried myself to sleep and mornings when getting out of bed felt almost impossible. There were days when depression sat on me like a weight and anxiety made every unknown feel bigger. There were times when the pain was so excruciating that I found myself thinking maybe death would be easier. I thought that if I were not here, my children would not have to keep living through this trauma with me.

But every time that thought tried to settle in, I would think about my children and the trauma of losing me. I knew that would wound them even more deeply. So they became enough. On those darkest days, they became my "why." They became enough to keep me here when I felt like I could not see light anywhere ahead of me.

With God as my foundation, my children, my family, and a whole lot of therapy, I made it through. I am battered and bruised, but I am here. Making my mental health a priority did not erase the pain, but it made a real difference in how I survived it.

Living with illness while also trying to hold everything together for my children often felt impossible. I was not just carrying my own pain; I was carrying the emotional labor of motherhood too. I was trying to protect my children while trying to show up from a place of depletion. That kind of split is exhausting.

What helped was honesty. It was not telling every person every detail, but being honest with myself, with God, and with the people closest to me. Admitting "I'm not okay" was freeing. Once I stopped pretending I was managing better than I was, other people could finally meet me where I truly was. They prayed with me, sat with me, and checked in on me.

The truth is that mental health is health. Ignoring it does not make you stronger; it only makes the burden heavier. My mind deserves care just as much as my body. Healing, in all its forms, often begins the moment we stop pretending we can carry everything alone.

Struggle

Depression and anxiety shadowed nearly every diagnosis. They were fed by grief, trauma, fear, and the constant uncertainty of not knowing what would happen next. Losing my stepmother shattered something deep in me, and before I could truly grieve her, I was thrown into survival mode. The unpredictability of flare-ups made planning difficult, and the fear of not being here for my children often became unbearable.

Insight

I learned that mental health is health. Ignoring my emotional pain did not make me stronger; it made me more fragile. Naming my grief, leaning into faith, and getting serious about therapy helped me survive some of the darkest days of my life. I also learned that on certain days, survival itself is holy work. When everything felt too dark, my children became enough.

Lesson

Tending to your mind is just as critical as tending to your body. Pain, grief, trauma, and fear can all live alongside chronic illness, and pretending otherwise only deepens the wound. Healing begins when we tell the truth about what we are carrying and let help meet us there.

Guidance

A few things that helped me care for my mental health:

- Seek therapy without shame. It is a tool rather than a weakness.
- Build mental health check-ins into your care routine just like medical appointments.
- Practice grounding tools such as prayer, journaling, deep breathing, or worship.

- Be honest with at least one trusted person when you are not okay.
- If you are spiraling, narrow the day down to one goal: survive today.
- Let your children, your faith, and your community remind you why your life matters.
- Remember that asking for help is not failure. It is wisdom and an act of strength.

CHAPTER 17

Faith & Resilience

When people ask me how I have survived everything I have faced, the blood clots, the surgeries, the strokes, the endless appointments, the uncertainty, the pain, and the exhaustion, my answer is simple: my faith. Without it, I do not know that I would have made it through the darkest seasons of my life. Faith has been my anchor.

But my walk with Christ did not begin in sickness. Faith had been part of my life long before my body became a battlefield. I grew up in the Catholic Church, served as an altar girl, and for a time I even wanted to become a nun like Mother Teresa. Even as a child, I was drawn to a life of devotion, sacrifice, and service. When illness came, I was not meeting God for the first time. I was returning to the One who had always been there, even if my journey with Him was about to deepen in a way I never expected.

In hospital rooms, when monitors beeped and doctors spoke in cautious tones, I prayed. In the nights when pain kept me awake and fear sat heavy on my chest, I prayed. In the moments when I felt alone, confused, or too tired to think clearly, I held on to the truth that God had not left me, even if I could not always make sense of what He was allowing me to walk through.

I clung to verses like Isaiah 41:10: "Fear thou not; for I am with thee: be not dismayed; for I am thy God." In seasons where my body felt fragile and my future uncertain, that promise became something I leaned on with everything I had.

But faith, for me, has never been about pretending. It has never meant smiling through suffering and acting like pain does not hurt. It has never meant having all the right words or always feeling spiritually strong. Sometimes faith looked strong, and sometimes it looked shaky. Sometimes it looked like worship, and sometimes it looked like tears. Sometimes it looked like silence and simply trying to survive the hour.

That is something I think is important to say, because too often people talk about faith as if it means never doubting, never struggling, and never feeling angry or weary. But my faith journey through illness has not been that polished. It has been real. It has been messy. It has been full of hope and questions living side by side.

There were times I trusted God deeply, and there were times I questioned everything. I did not question Him because I stopped believing, but because suffering has a way of forcing hard questions to the surface. How much can one person carry? Why does the body become a battlefield? Why does survival come at such a cost? These questions do not make faith weaker. They make it honest.

I had to learn that honesty belongs in my relationship with God too. There were moments when all I had was a whispered prayer, and moments when all I could say was, "Lord, help me." Somehow, even that was enough.

During one of the hardest seasons of my illness, I spoke to God with a level of surrender I had never known before. I told Him that if He got me through, I would give my life completely to Him. That was not a polished church prayer. It was the cry of a woman in pain who knew she needed God in a deeper way.

And then came a night I will never forget. It was my cousin's birthday party. I had not planned on going, but I decided to stop by just for the cake cutting. Somehow, I ended up staying until four o'clock in the morning. When I got to my car, a wave of emotion came over me so suddenly and so strongly that I could not hold it back. I sat there and cried like a baby for almost two hours.

It was as if something inside me had broken open. Around six o'clock that morning, I called my friend Joan and told her that I needed to get baptized right away. After taking baptism classes for two weeks, I was finally baptized, and I have never looked back.

That moment was not the beginning of my faith, but it was the beginning of a deeper surrender. It marked a new chapter in my walk with Christ, one where my faith became more than tradition. It became personal. It became the place where I laid my whole life down before God and said, "I am Yours."

God does not require a performance. He does not need me to sound strong in order to hold me up. He meets me in the truth of where I am, in the fear, the confusion, the grief, and the moments when all I have left is a fragile kind of faith that can barely lift its head. He has met me there over and over again.

There were scriptures that anchored me in ways I cannot fully explain. Some verses stopped being things I had merely heard in church and became lifelines. "The Lord is nigh unto them that are of a broken heart" (Psalm 34:18). "My grace is sufficient for thee: for my strength is made perfect in weakness" (2 Corinthians 12:9). When your body is failing you, you need truth strong enough to hold you when your emotions cannot.

Faith also gave me a lens through which to see resilience differently. Before illness, I might have thought resilience meant being strong all the time or never crying. But this journey taught me otherwise. Resilience is not pretending nothing hurts. It is not performing strength for other people or denying grief.

Real resilience is quieter than that. It is getting back up after being knocked down. It is taking the next breath when the last one felt heavy. It is letting yourself cry and still deciding not to quit. It is finding a way to keep going even if the only progress you can make that day is surviving it.

Some of my resilience came from faith, and some of it came through the people faith placed around me. My children, Chad and Kaitlyn, reminded me every day that I had reasons to keep going. My church reminded me that I was covered in prayer. My community reminded me that I was not walking this road alone. Resilience rarely grows in isolation. It is the strength that comes from being held up by love and by people who keep showing up when life is hard.

I have had moments where resilience looked big, like changing doctors or demanding better care. But most of the time, resilience looked much smaller. It looked like getting out of bed, taking my medicine, going to therapy, or praying one sentence.

Chronic illness teaches you that small acts can be sacred. What looks ordinary to others can be monumental when your body is in pain and your spirit is tired. Getting through the day can be an act of resilience. Asking for help can be an act of courage. Continuing to believe that your life still has meaning can be an act of holy resistance.

Faith and resilience have carried me side by side. Faith gives me hope, while resilience gives me movement. Faith reminds me who God is, and resilience reminds me to keep putting one foot in front of the other. Together, they have become the lifeline that has pulled me forward again and again.

I also had to learn that falling apart did not mean I had failed. It meant I was human, and by God's grace, I did not stay there forever. There were seasons when I felt broken and the grief sat heavy on me. There were seasons when faith did not feel triumphant. It felt thin, quiet, and fragile. But even then, something in me kept reaching toward God. Sometimes I reached with confidence, sometimes with desperation, and sometimes with no words at all. Resilience is often built in the reaching.

If there is one thing I want people to understand, it is that resilience is not the absence of struggle. It is what gets built inside the struggle. It is proof that by the grace of God, difficulty did not get the final word.

Faith is not always loud. Sometimes it is simply staying open to hope when everything in your life would tempt you to close. It is trusting that even if you cannot yet see the full picture, God still does. Jeremiah 29:11 took on a different meaning for me. It was not a shallow promise that life would be easy, but a reminder that God still had a purpose for me even when my life looked nothing like I thought it would.

Illness changed my life, but it did not erase my calling. Pain interrupted things, but it did not cancel my purpose. The same God who held me in hospital rooms and through surgeries is the same God who helped me keep going when I wanted to stop. Faith did not remove the struggle, but it gave me something steady inside it. Resilience did not make me superhuman. It made me willing to keep rising, even if slowly.

So when people say, "You are so strong," I understand what they mean. But what I know is this: I have been held. I have been carried. I have been strengthened in places where I had nothing left.

Resilience does not mean you never fall. It means you rise, even if it takes time. It means you keep reaching, even if your hands are shaking. It means you lean on your faith, your people, and your God, and trust that even in the struggle, grace is still holding you together.

Struggle

Faith did not make me immune to despair. There were times I doubted and times I felt worn thin. I wrestled with how a loving God could allow such relentless suffering. Chronic illness brought not only physical pain but spiritual questions too. It tested my trust, my hope, and my understanding of strength.

Insight

I learned that resilience is not about never breaking. It is about bending without being destroyed. I also learned that faith does not require perfection. It can coexist with grief, questions, and honest struggle. God met me not only in my strength, but in my weakness too.

Lesson

Resilience is built not in the absence of hardship, but in the practice of hope through it. Faith does not always remove the pain, but it can steady you inside it.

Guidance

A few things that helped anchor me:

- Let your faith be honest. God can handle your questions and your grief.
- Keep simple spiritual practices close, such as prayer, scripture, or worship.
- Do not measure your faith by how polished it looks. Sometimes a whispered "Lord, help me" is enough.
- Let community support your resilience through prayer and presence.

- Remember that small acts of endurance count. Getting through the day is holy work.
- When you cannot see the light clearly, borrow hope from what God has already brought you through.
- You do not have to be unshaken to be faithful. Sometimes faith looks like trembling and still holding on.

CHAPTER 18

Letters to My Children

If there is one thing this journey has taught me more than anything else, it is that love can carry a person through almost anything. When I think about the love that has carried me most, I think about my children.

Chad and Kaitlyn, you have both been woven into this story in ways that are impossible to separate from who I am. Every diagnosis, every hospital stay, every hard season, and every time I had to fight to keep going, the two of you were part of the reason I did.

This chapter is for you. It is not because I have found the perfect words for everything this journey has cost us, but because I want what is in my heart to live on paper. I want you to know what you have meant to me and what I have seen in you. I want you to know that even in the middle of so much pain, the two of you have been among the greatest gifts of my life.

To Chad

Chad, you are my firstborn. There is something so special about a firstborn child. In many ways, we grew up together. I became a mother with you, and I became myself in deeper ways because of you. There has always been a bond between us that is hard to fully explain. It is love, yes, but it is also history. It is the shared growing pains of life and the way we learned each other through the years. It is that quiet understanding that comes from having been there from the beginning.

You have always held such a special place in my heart. When my health began to spiral, you stepped into a role that no child should have to carry so young. Instead of being free to focus only on your own life, your own path, and your own beginning, you came home. You helped take care of me and your baby sister. You became steady when life felt shaky. You became dependable when everything else felt uncertain. You loved us in action, not just in words.

You took care of Kaitlyn like she was your own child. You watched over her, protected her, and carried a responsibility that was heavy. You did it with a grace that still humbles me. You were the big brother and son I had prayed for even before I fully knew how much I would need the exact heart God gave you.

I need you to know that I see that. I see the sacrifice. I see the quiet weight you carried. I see the way you put us first over and over again.

And I also need you to know this: I carry guilt over how much this illness asked of you. Even now, there are times when I look at you and wonder how different your life might have been if you had not had to carry so much so early. While other young men were free to move through life more lightly, you were helping keep this family standing. That is a heavy thing for a mother to hold. But alongside that guilt, I hold so much pride.

Even though you tell me all the time that you want to be here and that you want to help, I still feel the ache of it. I cannot help but wonder whether my illness asked too much of you. I cannot help but feel the sorrow of knowing that while other young men were free to move through life more lightly, you were helping keep this family standing.

That is a heavy thing for a mother to hold. Yet what I hold alongside that guilt is pride. So much pride. The way you have loved us says everything about the kind of man you are: quietly strong, loyal, protective, and dependable. You have loved this family with your whole life, and that kind of love is rare.

Still, I want this said clearly on these pages: I want you to live. I want you to really live. I want you to build your own life fully and boldly without feeling like your only role is to carry everyone else. I want you to dream big, take chances, and experience the fullness of the life God has for you. Loving us well should not mean putting your whole future on pause forever.

You have given so much, and I want life to give back to you too. Thank you for being my son. Thank you for being my strength on days when I had none. Thank you for being the kind of man who loves deeply, serves quietly, and shows up consistently. No matter where life takes you, you will always be my first baby, my heart, and one of the greatest answered prayers of my life.

To Kaitlyn

Kaitlyn, my girl, my mini-me, my heart, my bestie. There are not enough words for what you mean to me. You came into my life wrapped in both joy and survival. Even before you were born, we were already fighting for our lives together. In so many ways, that has shaped the bond we share. You have been part of my story from the very beginning of this battle, but never just as a witness. You have been one of the brightest lights in it.

You are seventeen now. Even writing that makes me stop and breathe for a moment because I can still see the baby girl I was dressing with one good arm while trying not to panic. I can still see the little girl who had to grow up around hospitals, appointments, and a mother whose body was often in crisis. Now here you are on the edge of leaving for college, standing in your own becoming.

If I am honest, I am struggling with letting you go. I know that is part of motherhood. I know children are meant to grow, stretch, and leave the nest to discover who they are in the world. I want that for you. I want every beautiful thing for you. But you have been so close to me for so long that the thought of that distance tugs hard at my heart.

When you were five years old, you were diagnosed with severe separation anxiety. Truthfully, the way you still stalk me sometimes makes me wonder whether you ever fully got over it. That makes me laugh even as it makes me emotional. You check my location when I am out. You give me hugs throughout the day. You tell me all the time how much you love me. Every time you do, some part of me is healed by it.

Watching you become who you are has been one of the greatest joys of my life. Even in a life that has held so much pain, you are one of the clearest proofs that beauty still grows. You are an award-winning poet and the current Poet Laureate of our city. You are an actress, a singer, and an amazing writer. You have owned your own business since you were eight years old. You have used your gifts to serve your community through events for kids, families, and seniors. You are not just talented; you are compassionate.

I am in awe of you. One of the reasons I push so hard and keep fighting through the pain is because I want to see you live and thrive. I want to see you blossom into the woman I already know you are becoming.

I have done my best to teach you how to advocate, not just for yourself, but for people who do not have a voice. I see in you the heart of a warrior. I know that whatever you do in life, you will do it with authenticity, courage, and purpose. I know you will be great because your spirit is strong.

More than anything, I pray every day that you will continue to grow in your faith. I want you rooted in God. I want you to know who you are and whose you are. As you prepare to leave for college, I want you to carry this with you: you do not have to stop being tender to be strong. You do not have to stop being loving to be ambitious. Take your whole heart with you, your words, your gifts, your creativity, and your faith. Know that no matter how far you go, there will always be a place in me that is yours alone.

To Both of You

I need both of you to know this: I have loved you with everything in me. Not perfectly, but fiercely, deeply, and honestly. The journey we have walked together has not been easy. Illness touched all of us. It changed our family life and brought fear into our home at times. It forced all of us to grow in ways we probably would not have chosen.

But it also revealed who we are. Who you both are is extraordinary. We may not have a lot of money. I have not been able to work the way I once might have dreamed. There have been real limits and sacrifices. But we are rich in other ways: rich in love, resilience, faith, loyalty, and the kind of connection money cannot buy.

I love you both with all that I have. You have been my why. That truth has kept me going every single day. You became one of the clearest reasons I stayed and kept fighting.

You became enough. You became the reason I stayed and the reason I kept fighting. In my eyes, you are perfect. You are perfect because you are mine and because the love God placed in this family has been one of the most beautiful gifts of my life.

If there is anything I hope you carry from this journey, it is not just the memory of what was hard. I hope you carry the memory of what held us. Love held us. Faith held us. Community held us. Grace held us. And somehow, through it all, we held each other too.

I want you to know that I am proud of you, not just for what you do, but for who you are. If I have one prayer for your future, it is this: that you both live big, beautiful, purpose-filled lives. That you love deeply without losing yourselves. That you know your worth and walk in faith. And that even when life is hard, you remember what this family has already proven: we bend, we grieve, and we struggle, but by the grace of God, we keep going.

With all my love,
Mom

Struggle

One of the deepest struggles of this journey has been knowing that my illness did not only affect me. It touched my children too. Chad had to grow up faster than he should have. Kaitlyn had to live with a mother whose health could change in an instant. That reality has brought me both gratitude for their love and guilt for what this road has required of them.

Insight

Love has been one of the greatest forms of strength in my life. My children did not just witness my journey. They became part of what kept me alive inside it. Through them, I learned that even when illness changes the shape of life, it does not have the power to remove its deepest meaning.

Lesson

The people you love can become part of your survival story. Sometimes the greatest legacy pain leaves behind is not only what it took, but what it taught your family about love, resilience, service, and staying power.

Guidance

If illness has affected your family, remember this:

- Tell your children the truth in age-appropriate ways.
- Let love be spoken out loud often.
- Do not assume they know how much they matter to you; say it.
- Make room for both gratitude and grief.
- Let your family's story include not only pain, but purpose.

Love does not erase hardship, but it can carry you through it.

CHAPTER 19

A New Purpose

Chronic illness stripped away so much of the life I thought I would have. It took my independence in ways I never expected. It interrupted dreams I had for my career, my future, and the life I imagined I would be living. It took my sense of normalcy and replaced it with uncertainty. It took ease and replaced it with effort.

For a long time, all I could see was what had been lost. I felt the loss of freedom, the loss of energy, and the loss of the life I had expected to unfold. There were seasons when that grief felt louder than anything else. Long hospital stays and endless appointments made it hard to imagine that anything good could grow out of so much disruption.

At first, I did not see purpose; I saw pain. But over time, something began to shift. It happened slowly, like light returning after a very long night. I began to realize that while illness had changed my path, it had not ended it. It had redirected me.

There is a difference between an ending and a redirection, even though they can feel the same in the beginning. Sometimes God does not end the story. Sometimes He rewrites the assignment.

The more I learned to speak up for myself, the more I wanted to help other people do the same. I knew what it felt like to be dismissed, overlooked, and made to feel small. Once you have lived through enough pain, you start to recognize how powerful it is to become the kind of person you once needed.

Out of that passion, new seeds were planted. One of the most meaningful was **Kaitlyn Cares**, which I co-founded with my daughter. It came from a desire to pour back into the same community that had poured so much into us during our hardest seasons. There is something especially sacred to me about building that with Kaitlyn. She was not only part of my struggle. She became part of my purpose.

I still remember Kaitlyn designing her first T-shirt. We put the shirts on Amazon, and when she got her first check, I asked her what she wanted to do with the money. She said she wanted to do something for the children in the community at the library. Because Kaitlyn has always loved breakfast, we decided to turn it into a breakfast event.

That is how our annual **Pancakes and Pajamas** was born. The amount she earned was not much, but the point was her heart. For years, Chad and I have funded these events out of our own pockets with the help of a few faithful friends. People see the event itself, but they do not always see the planning, the stretching, and the quiet commitment to keep pouring even when your own resources are limited.

Our annual Pancakes and Pajamas has become a special moment of warmth and togetherness. We also created the **Teens to Seniors Breakfast**, now in its fourth year, to bridge the gap between generations in a world that too often keeps them separate. Then there is **Echoes of Expression Poetry Slam**, Kaitlyn's poetry event for teens, and **Boss Up Through Entrepreneurship**, where she teaches other teens how to start their own businesses. Every event we put on includes food or snack packs because food insecurity is real in our community. We do not just want people to leave inspired. We want them to leave helped.

Furthermore, my son Chad and I founded **KindRoot Wellness**, a wellness app and website for people living with chronic illness. It came from wanting to create a daily companion for people walking through uncertainty and helps people navigate the healthcare system while learning how to advocate for themselves.

That is what purpose does: it takes pain and makes it useful. It takes what tried to break you and lets it become a doorway for someone else. That does not mean the pain was worth it or that I would have chosen this road, but it does mean that God has a way of pulling something living out of places that once felt dead.

These were not just projects. They were lifelines. They gave me a reason to get out of bed on the hard days and reminded me that survival could still become impact.

Illness closed one chapter of my life. There were dreams that had to die and versions of myself I had to grieve. But illness also opened another chapter rooted in advocacy, service, and love. It reminded me that my story was not over just because it changed. In that purpose, I found something illness could never take away: hope.

I mean the kind of hope that has walked through fire and still believes something good can rise. That is the hope I live in now, and it is part of my purpose too.

Struggle

At first, all I could see was what illness had taken from me. My independence, my plans, and my dreams were all reshaped. It was hard not to measure life by loss. In the beginning, purpose felt very far away.

Insight

I learned that redirection is not the same as destruction. Illness changed my path, but it did not erase my value. Purpose did not arrive by denying the pain; it came by allowing the pain to shape me into someone who could serve and advocate for others.

Lesson

Pain can become purpose when we refuse to let it be the final word. What tries to silence you can also become the place where your voice grows strongest.

Guidance

A few things I learned about finding purpose after pain:

- Do not rush purpose. Let it grow honestly from what you have lived through.
- Pay attention to what breaks your heart. Often purpose lives nearby.
- Ask yourself: *What have I learned that could help someone else?*
- Start small. Purpose often begins as one act of service.
- Let your pain deepen your empathy rather than harden your heart.
- Remember that purpose and grief can exist at the same time.

Your story may have changed, but it still has purpose.

CHAPTER 20

Your Turn to Advocate

By now, you have walked with me through the twists and turns of my journey. You have seen the emergencies, the dismissals, the long nights, and the surgeries. You have witnessed the grief, the breakthroughs, the moments that broke me, and the lessons that reshaped how I see healthcare and how I see myself.

But this chapter is not about me. It is about you.

If there is one truth I hope you carry from these pages, it is this: you are your own best advocate. No one else lives in your body. No one else feels your pain, your symptoms, or your intuition when something is wrong. Doctors, nurses, therapists, and specialists may be experts in medicine, but you are the expert in your own life.

That matters. It matters in the exam room, the emergency room, the pharmacy, and the hospital. It matters every time your body tells you something is wrong and the world around you is not moving fast enough to catch up.

Advocacy does not require a degree or perfect words. It does not require boldness every single time. It begins with simple steps. It begins the moment you decide that your life is worth paying attention to.

Keep a journal. Write down your symptoms, medications, side effects, questions, and test results. Small details today may become life saving information tomorrow. Ask questions, no matter how small or "silly" they may feel. If you do not understand something, you have the right to ask until it makes sense. If the room is moving too fast, slow it down.

Do not be afraid to change doctors. The right one will listen, partner with you, and respect you. The wrong one will drain you. You deserve better. Trust yourself. If something feels wrong, it probably deserves attention. Do not let anyone convince you that your instincts mean nothing.

Advocacy also means giving yourself grace. There will be days when you do not feel strong enough to fight or days when you are too tired to explain one more symptom. You do not have to do this perfectly. You just have to keep showing up for yourself again and again.

Some days advocacy is direct, and some days it is quiet. Some days it looks like asking ten questions, and some days it looks like one sentence: "Something is wrong, and I need you to listen." Some days it looks like going to the ER, and other days it looks like resting or asking for help because your body has reached its limit. That counts too.

Advocacy is not selfish. It does not only protect your body; it protects your future, your family, your peace of mind, and your dignity. When you speak up for yourself, you are often teaching other people how to value themselves too. Your children see it. Your family sees it. Your community sees it. Sometimes your courage becomes permission for someone else to use their voice too.

Your story can become a bridge. Your persistence can become a lifeline for someone else.

Still, I want to be honest. Advocacy is not easy. The system is intimidating and the stakes are high. There is always that temptation to go quiet, to not cause trouble, or to not be "too much." But silence costs more than discomfort.

Silence costs answers, clarity, and dignity. Sometimes, silence costs time you cannot afford to lose.

If you are wondering whether you really have it in you to advocate for yourself, let me tell you this: yes, you do. Maybe not all at once or in a polished way, but you do. You can write one question down. You can ask for clarification. You can say, "That does not match what I'm feeling." You can request a second opinion. You can ask that your concern be documented. Every time you do it, that muscle gets stronger.

I cannot promise the road ahead will be easy, but I can promise this: you are not powerless. You have wisdom, instincts, and every right to insist on the care you deserve. So take a breath. Write down your questions. Walk into that appointment with courage, even if it is shaky courage. Remember that what you are experiencing deserves attention. Now it is your turn to advocate.

Now, it is your turn to advocate.

Struggle

Advocacy feels daunting at first. The system is intimidating, the stakes are high, and fear can make silence look easier than speaking up. Many of us have been taught to be cooperative and undemanding even when our bodies are telling a very different story.

Insight

You do not have to know everything to advocate for yourself. Advocacy is a muscle that grows every time you use it.

Lesson

Use your story, your questions, and your voice.

Guidance

A few places to start:

- Keep a notebook or notes app with symptoms, medications, and questions.
- Bring your top three concerns into every appointment.
- Ask for explanations in plain language.
- Bring support if you need another set of ears or a steadier voice.
- Trust your instincts when something feels off.
- Ask for documentation when your concern is being minimized.
- Remember that you can leave providers who do not respect you.
- Keep going even if your advocacy starts small.

You do not have to become fearless. You just have to keep choosing not to disappear. We must never stop insisting on being seen.

CONCLUSION

Carrying Hope Forward

As I look back on the years since that morning when my arm first turned blue, I am struck by how much has changed and how much I have changed with it.

What began in fear, confusion, and crisis became a journey of resilience, faith, advocacy, and purpose. I never asked for chronic illness. I never asked for the hospital stays, the surgeries, the endless appointments, or the loneliness. I never asked for the pain, the dismissals that left me in tears, or a body that would become so unpredictable. I never asked for a life that would require so much fighting just to hold on to what others take for granted.

But I also never could have imagined the strength I would find along the way. I never imagined the wisdom that would grow out of suffering. I never imagined the depth of love, faith, and community that would carry me through the hardest seasons of my life. And I never imagined that this journey would uncover a new purpose within me.

This road has been about more than survival. It has been about learning how to live differently. It has been about learning how to fight, trust, speak, and believe differently. It has been about learning to see myself not only as a patient, but as an advocate. I am not only someone who suffers. I am someone who still has purpose. I am not only a woman carrying pain. I am a mother, a friend, a leader, and a woman still filled with hope.

The road has not been easy. And if I am honest, it still is not. There are still days when the pain is sharp and the fatigue feels unbearable. There are days when grief rises again. There are days when the weight of it all feels so heavy that giving up seems easier than trying one more time.

But on those days, I remind myself of every moment I have already made it through. I remind myself that God has carried me before, and He is carrying me still. I remind myself that resilience is not built only in grand, dramatic moments. It is built one breath, one decision, one prayer, one appointment, and one act of courage at a time. It is built every time we choose not to quit.

To you, dear reader, I want to leave this reminder: you are not powerless in your journey. Whether you are just beginning this road or have been walking it for years, what you are experiencing deserves attention. Your fight is worth it.

Carry forward the lessons from these pages. Keep your journal and ask your questions. Build your support circle and lean on your faith. Take care of your mental health and trust what your body is telling you. Never be afraid to walk away from care that does not honor your dignity.

Most of all, carry hope. I do not mean shallow hope or the kind that denies pain or pretends everything is fine. I mean the kind of hope that survives hard nights. The kind of hope that breathes through tears and keeps you reaching for tomorrow even when today is hard.

Hope is what steadies us. Hope is what helps us imagine life beyond this moment. Hope is what reminds us that no matter how fierce the struggle, there is still beauty, still grace, and still purpose woven through our lives.

This is not the end of my journey, and it may not be the end of yours either. But as we walk forward, may we do so knowing that we are stronger than we think, braver than we feel, and more resilient than we ever imagined. And may we never forget that even in the struggle, there is always room for grace.

My honest take: this version is cleaner because it trims the repeated "your voice matters / your body matters / your story matters" language and lets the conclusion sound more final, more mature, and less like another advocacy chapter.

Appendix
Simplified Book Edition

A concise, reader-friendly version of the support tools included in the companion packet.

This book appendix gives you a quick, clean overview of the tools. For full printable worksheets, trackers, and guided pages, use the separate appendix packet.

How to Use This Appendix

Living with chronic illness often means holding too much information at once. This simplified appendix is designed to make the essentials easier to find and easier to use. Think of it as a quick-reference version of the companion packet: enough to guide you, prepare you, and remind you what matters most when you are tired, overwhelmed, or trying to think clearly in a hard moment.

Start with the page that meets your immediate need. Some days that may be your symptom notes. Other days it may be your appointment questions, your emergency plan, or the simple reminder that your voice matters.

Contents

1. Symptom Tracker

Use this tool to capture what happened, when it started, how intense it felt, and what changed. A clear symptom record helps you notice patterns and communicate more precisely.

- Write down the date, time, and body area affected.
- Rate the pain or severity from 0 to 10.
- Note what you were doing before it started.
- Record what made it worse, what helped, and how long it lasted.
- If there was swelling, bruising, color change, numbness, or weakness, write that down too.

2. Medication Tracker

This page helps you keep a simple record of what you take and why. When medications change often, a written list protects you from confusion.

- List the medication name and dosage.
- Write what it is for in plain language.
- Track side effects you notice in real life, not just the ones on paper.
- Keep the prescribing doctor attached to each medication when possible.

3. Appointment Preparation Sheet

Appointments move quickly. This tool helps you walk in focused and leave with fewer loose ends.

- Write your main concern at the top.
- Choose your top three questions before the visit.
- Bring notes on new symptoms, medication concerns, or test requests.
- Decide what answer or next step you need before the appointment ends.

4. Questions to Ask Your Doctor

When your mind is tired, it helps to have a few steady questions ready.

- What are you ruling in?
- What are you ruling out?
- What happens if this test is negative?
- Can you explain that in plain English?
- Can you document this concern in my chart?

5. Medical History One-Page Summary

This is your quick-reference health snapshot. It is especially useful in emergencies, new appointments, or hospital visits.

- Include diagnoses, surgeries, allergies, major medications, and key doctors.
- Keep an emergency contact on the page.
- If you take a blood thinner or have a high-risk condition, make that easy to see.

6. Emergency Plan Sheet

In a true emergency, thinking gets harder. A plan reduces panic and saves time.

- Know who can take you to the ER.
- Know who can care for your children or update loved ones.
- List the hospital you prefer, if you have one.
- Include critical diagnoses, allergies, and urgent medications.

7. Support Circle Contact Sheet

Support is easier to use when it is organized. This page helps you match names to the kind of help each person can offer.

- List who can help with rides, meals, childcare, hospital visits, or prayer.
- Do not wait for crisis to figure out who is available.
- Specific support is easier to ask for and easier for others to give.

8. Hospital Bag Checklist

A small ready bag can make a chaotic hospital trip feel less chaotic.

- Keep your ID, insurance card, medication list, and phone charger ready.
- Add comfortable clothes, toiletries, and a notebook.
- If you wear glasses or use headphones, pack those too.

9. Complaint Letter Template

When a medical encounter causes harm, a written complaint can create a record and ask for accountability.

- State the date, provider, and location clearly.
- Describe what happened without overexplaining.
- Say why the care was harmful and what review you are requesting.
- Keep your tone calm, direct, and factual.

10. Patient Advocacy Reminders

Some truths are worth keeping close when you feel intimidated or exhausted.

- My pain is real.
- I know my body better than anyone else.

- I am allowed to ask questions and ask again.
- I am allowed to seek a second opinion.
- I am allowed to leave providers who do not respect me.

11. Grounding Tools for Hard Days

When fear spikes or your thoughts start running ahead of you, grounding helps bring you back to the next steady step.

- Take five slow breaths.
- Name five things you can see.
- Repeat one truth: I only have to survive today.
- Call or text one trusted person.
- Write down what feels hardest right now.

12. Resources

Use the companion packet for the full resource list with contact details. Inside the book, keep the categories in mind so you know where to turn first.

- Rare disease and undiagnosed condition support
- Patient advocacy and medical navigation
- Mental health and crisis support
- Women's health and Black women's health resources
- Condition-specific support

A Note to the Reader

You do not have to use every tool at once. Start with one page that helps you breathe a little easier, prepare a little better, or feel a little less alone. That is enough.

For full printable trackers, writing space, and worksheet-style versions of these pages, use the companion appendix packet.

www.ingramcontent.com/pod-product-compliance
Lightning Source LLC
LaVergne TN
LVHW010619100826
845148LV00014B/3036

* 9 7 9 8 2 3 4 0 5 6 6 0 3 *